Testimonial

This is a wonderful and important book. These fascinating, inspiring stories about the work of nurse practitioners jump off the page with intelligence and energy. Read them for enjoyment, but also, read them to understand how NPs have the potential to improve health care efficiency, universal access, provision of primary care, management of chronic illness, and lengthy wait times. With more NPs, we'll be a healthier and thus happier, society.

Tilda Shalof, RN, BScN, CCNC (c)

Bestselling author of *A Nurse's Story* and *Bringing it Home*.

No One Left Behind

How Nurse Practitioners Are Changing The Canadian Health Care System

Claudia Mariano

MSc, NP-PHC, CDE

FriesenPress
Suite 300 - 990 Fort St
Victoria, BC, Canada, V8V 3K2
www.friesenpress.com

First Edition — 2015

While the stories in "No One Left Behind" are based on real events, patient names or other identifying details have been changed to protect the privacy and anonymity of the individuals and facilities involved.

ISBN
978-1-4602-6320-4 (Hardcover)
978-1-4602-6321-1 (Paperback)
978-1-4602-6322-8 (eBook)

1. Medical, Family & General Practice

Distributed to the trade by The Ingram Book Company

Table of Contents

To my husband Louis,
and my parents
Anneliese and Egon Weidenborner,
For always believing in me

Foreword

This book is about real patients and the real Nurse Practitioners who care for them. Stories about health care are in the news every day, whether it's about the safety risks associated with medications or the shortage of services for seniors or threats to funding. But the relationship between the health care provider and the patient is often seen as a private experience cloaked in secrecy and mystified by medical jargon.

Through this remarkable compilation of stories, Claudia Mariano helps to lift the veil on this private world by inviting the reader to share in the intimate relationships that form between patients and Nurse Practitioners. This book shines a light on the real life experiences of patients and the world they live in as seen through the eyes of the Canadian Nurse Practitioners who care about them and for them.

The stories you will read are both heart-wrenching and soul-affirming. They give testimony to the frailty of the human body and the strength of the human spirit. Challenges and health problems are met with resilience and resourcefulness. You will be struck by the courage and compassion that helps to define humanity.

Nurse Practitioners have the privilege of being with people during life-changing events and throughout their lifespan. These wonderful stories that are told by Nurse Practitioners highlight how having expertise at a molecular level is not enough. People are more than their illness, they are more than their addiction, and yes, they come into a clinic with more than one problem. You will see how Nurse Practitioners through compassion and courage really have become game-changers. In each chapter you will meet ordinary people providing extraordinary care in an attempt to make life better.

If you have encountered health problems, you will be able to relate. If you are thinking of becoming a health care professional, you will be inspired. And if you have ever found yourself thinking about how to turn our illness-treatment system into a health care system, you will be motivated to take action. Finally, you will be left with the thought: doesn't every Canadian deserve the exceptional care that Nurse Practitioners provide?

Theresa Agnew BA (SDS), NP-PHC
Executive Director
Nurse Practitioners' Association of Ontario

Introduction

You're a what? I think I've heard of that, you can prescribe stuff, right? Why didn't you become a doctor? So you're kind of a super-nurse . . . . These are just some of the comments I've received over the years when I tell people I'm a nurse practitioner (NP). In some ways – as the rules and regulations governing NPs have changed over the years – it's been easier to talk about my work in terms of what I *can't* do, rather than what I *can*. Historically, registered nurses have worked in expanded roles for decades, especially in remote parts of Canada where there is a chronic lack of access to health care. As outpost nurses, they often worked in expanded roles, taking on activities that were traditionally within the medical realm. These early outpost nurses were the predecessors of today's NPs, particularly in primary health care. During the 1960s and 1970s, the introduction of universal publically funded medical insurance, an increased emphasis on primary health care, and a perceived physician shortage were driving forces for the full implementation of a distinct NP role[1]

1 For a full review of the historical development of the nurse practitioner role in Canada, the reader is directed to Nursing Leadership, (23), December 2010, Special Issue.

When the first Canadian NP education program began in Hamilton, Ontario in the early 1970s, the idea was to educate experienced registered nurses to enable them to see patients independently, diagnose illness, prescribe medications, and order the necessary tests. NP education programs have evolved over the years to keep up with the demands of clinical practice in a rapidly changing health care environment, and focus on providing experienced registered nurses with the education necessary to independently assess patients, diagnose illness, prescribe medications, and order laboratory and diagnostic testing. While this overlaps with the role of physicians, you will discover that NPs utilize a solid nursing foundation, which focuses on wellness, teaching, and advocacy for their patients, regardless of where they live or what ails them.

This didn't happen all at once. Current health care policies are firmly entrenched in a model of health care based on hospitals and solo physicians providing care. NPs don't fit well with these policies, and changing them is a battle in itself. And so the journey of NPs in Canada is a decades-long story filled with politics, detours, lost ground, standing our ground, baby steps, courage—and always knowing that our patients and communities are at the heart of our work. Where once there were just a few scattered NPs working alone to provide the best health care possible to Canadians in isolated areas of our country, now there are over 3200 working in every province and territory across the country, with over 2600 practising in Ontario. From community clinics to hospitals, from emergency departments to long-term care facilities, NPs are providing outstanding care to patients across the country, working with teams of health care professionals in all settings to ensure the best possible outcomes for our patients.

As the role of the NP has changed over the years, the answer to the question "what do nurse practitioners do?" has changed as well. And who better answer that question than the NPs themselves. Throughout these pages, you will learn about the real work of Canadian NPs, work that involves joy and sorrow, deep nursing knowledge and skill, and even deeper compassion and courage. Though all of the experiences themselves are true, each writer has changed the identity of their patients to protect their privacy.

Much has changed since the first NPs entered the Canadian health care scene over forty years ago. Knowledge and attitudes have evolved. While the accounts of the early days are not the experiences of today (for patients or for NPs), they are stories which describe the road we have travelled to get here. They are not intended to be a criticism of any particular organization or individual, but to allow NPs to tell their stories. In the future, as our role continues to evolve, the one constant will be our desire to fight for our patients.

In the Heat of the Day

Claudia Mariano MSc, NP-PHC, CDE

As I entered the small apartment, my lungs immediately protested the forced inhalation of the acrid air, and I gasped. The heat was stifling, even for August, and beads of sweat had already begun to form across my brow. The little boy, no more than eight or nine years old, was lying on a mattress in the middle of the room, his mother kneeling beside him, wiping his forehead with a damp cloth. Most of his upper body was encased in a spica cast, holding his arm away from his body. That morning, the boy's father had called the community health centre where I worked, and where the family received their health care. His son had a fever, and they couldn't get him to the clinic because of the cast, and they had no car. He had pleaded for someone to come out to their home to check on their son.

As I wasn't familiar with the family, I had reviewed the boy's chart after agreeing to the receptionist's request to squeeze in a home visit. I discovered that they had recently moved to this rental apartment, after arriving from Eastern Europe six months earlier. The boy, Daniil, who had recently had shoulder surgery for a congenital dislocation, had developed a fever overnight and wasn't drinking very much. Having reviewed my patient appointments for the day, I asked the receptionist to call the family earlier that morning to let them know that I would be at their home by noon. Given that there was no other time available to me, I would have to make the visit during my lunch hour. Not knowing what to expect, I reviewed the contents of the home visit bag, and threw in a prescription pad, just in case.

Now, having just walked up a narrow flight of stairs into the apartment, I felt a pang of guilt. I had driven and walked past these storefront apartments dozens of times over the years, shopping in the trendy stores below, blissfully unaware of how the people above me were living. This couldn't even be called an apartment. Just two rooms, the smaller one housing a tiny galley kitchen, and the larger room I was standing in. There were no windows, the only entrance was the staircase from the street below. The single light bulb hanging in the middle of the ceiling cast dark shadows, which only etched the deep creases further into the faces of the man and woman standing over the little boy on the mattress. The walls of the tiny room were stacked with boxes holding clothes and dishware.

The boy's father thanked me for coming and then went on to tell me that his son was not well, and as a result, had been unable to eat or drink. In halting English he pleaded for my help, while gesturing to the sick boy on the mattress.

I wiped the sweat from my forehead with the back of my hand, then knelt on the floor beside the mattress. As I opened the house call bag and took out the hand sanitizer, I smiled reassuringly at Daniil and his worried parents and introduced myself as the NP from the clinic they attended.

Looking down at the boy, I asked how much he had to drink that day. Daniil's eyes were half-open beneath a mass of dark hair; his lips were peeling, and his parents confirmed that he had taken only a few sips of water. Daniil's mother continued to bathe her son's forehead with water as I took out the thermometer and held it in his ear. I spoke calmly to the boy, attempting to reassure him and his parents that he was going to be okay. His eyes opened wider at the sound of my voice, but I was growing increasingly concerned at his lack of response. The thermometer beeped and I glanced at the reading, confirming what I already suspected. He was feverish . . . his little body trying desperately to ward off unseen invaders, and with the cumbersome cast and the heat, I could only imagine how much pain he was in.

I took out my stethoscope and placed it on Daniil's chest. His heartbeat, though regular, was too rapid for my liking, and I frowned slightly. As I wrapped the blood pressure cuff around his arm, I made attempts to get more information from his parents, which would allow me to understand the boy's medical history. *What medications was he taking? When had he been discharged from hospital? When was he to see the surgeon for follow up and removal of the cast?*

As I released the air from the blood pressure cuff Daniil stirred and attempted to move, the bulky cast preventing him from changing position. He whimpered and his mother moved her face closer to his, singing softly to him.

I motioned to Daniil's father to kneel beside me, and together we gently turned him onto his good side. Then I gestured to his mother to switch places with me, and I moved to the other side to examine Daniil's back. I suspected he might be developing a bedsore from the heat and pressure of not being able to change position. With his back now exposed, I gently lowered the band of his underwear and found what I feared – a red, open, oozing spot at the base of his spine. This would quickly become infected, if it wasn't already.

I motioned for Daniil's parents to look, and they craned their necks to see. His mother moaned when she saw the scourge on her son's flesh, and tears streamed down her face.

Having listened to her pleas, I swallowed hard and stomped down on the rage that was building inside me. I told myself to keep cool and then informed the boy's parents that I was going to dress the wound. I reached into my home visit bag for the dressing supplies, and quickly cleansed the wound with saline, then applied gauze and a large adhesive bandage. The extra padding would help alleviate the pressure until he could be assessed further in hospital. I knew there was no point writing a prescription for antibiotics, he needed to go to the hospital and be assessed for possible sepsis, a potentially life-threatening complication of infection.

I told his parents that he had an infection and that he needed to go back to the hospital. I asked if there was anyone who could drive him there, and Daniil's father shook his head to reveal what I already knew, so I called for an ambulance, giving the operator details of the boy's condition and that I suspected symptoms of sepsis.

As Daniil's parents gathered up a few belongings in preparation for another trip to the hospital, I asked for the phone number of the landlord, offering to contact him to advise him of what had happened. Daniil's father handed me a scrap of paper with a name and phone number scribbled on it, and I grabbed a pen from my pocket and wrote the number on my sweaty palm, praying it wouldn't smudge before I could make the call.

I remember feeling a wave of relief as I heard the wail of the siren as the ambulance made its approach. I informed the family that I would go downstairs to let the paramedics know which room to go to. I also needed to get away from the stifling heat and into the fresh air. I was angry. This family was living in what amounted to nothing more than a closet, and someone was actually taking money from them for it.

I waved at the ambulance as it pulled over to the curb in front of me. As the two paramedics began to remove the stretcher from the back of the vehicle, I gave them a summary of Daniil's history and current status, as well as my contact information from the clinic. I waited until the ambulance left with Daniil and his parents safely inside and, having already extracted a promise from Daniil's father to let me know the next day how his son was doing, I headed back to the clinic to deal with the landlord.

I squinted at the numbers scribbled on my palm as I punched them angrily into the phone. A man picked up on the third ring, and I struggled to remain professional as I introduced myself and then proceeded to voice my concerns on the living conditions of the family's apartment. I told the landlord that there was no window, no smoke alarm and only one entrance, and that in the event of a fire, there would be no way out if the door was blocked.

The man snorted into the phone, informing me that the fire department had already made their inspections and that everything was fine and legal.

I told him that was great to hear, however, I would request that they stop by once again just to double check.

After a prolonged silence, the landlord finally agreed to move the family to a bigger unit, although I could tell he was angry. Nevertheless, I thanked him for doing the right thing, although he slammed the phone down before I was able to finish what I was saying.

I sighed and turned my attention back to the computer screen to complete my documentation of the visit. I had already asked the Social Worker on our team to follow up with the family upon discharge from the hospital, to ensure they had adequate housing and the landlord was good to his word. Stethoscopes and medicine could only fix so much. My stomach rumbled as I glanced at my schedule on the computer screen and noticed my next patient had arrived.

It was going to be a long afternoon.

A Second Chance

Kate Burkholder MN, NP

It was a cold, gloomy, January day when Joey entered my office. His previous provider had retired and he had not seen anyone for health care for some time. He walked in slumped over, head bent, looking down, and avoided any eye contact. His old jacket and ball cap did not seem warm enough for the temperatures outside; however, he claimed that the walk had warmed him up.

Joey went on to give me some details of his life: he lived alone and didn't have a job; in fact, by his own admission, he couldn't read or write. We talked more about his life in general and his medical history. Joey was an albino, which he said caused a lot of grief, and on one occasion when he was seventeen, he had been beaten up and left to die, all because they didn't like the look of him. Hearing this sad account and the vile acts that others could place on a human being and how their future could be affected, upset me to the core.

In a small town you rely on friends, family, and co-workers as your supports for guidance, caring and a listening ear. I had immediately taken a liking to this man in front of me. He had not had any support for years. In a town that did not have any local transport or taxi service, it meant if you did not own your own car then you would be reliant on others. But nobody had ever stopped to ask Joey if he wanted to go into town or whether he required any food or any other service. His social isolation was immense.

He cried as he told me how all he wanted was a second chance. He smoked at least a packet of cigarettes a day, while drinking six cans of beer to make himself feel better. However, having admitted he felt no better and that his nerves were really bad, he informed me that he found it difficult to rely on anybody for help. We talked about the small, gradual steps that were needed toward change and, after he looked at me and raised a faint smile, he told me that he would try.

Over the first few visits, we laughed a lot. Joey liked to laugh, joke and giggle, and we cried together too, at the inequality of life and the disparity many people have to live with. I had come to find over a very short time that he had a remarkable sense of humour and a huge heart. However, I could see that there were many other challenges ahead.

As a new NP, I thought about the social determinants of health, chronic diseases, and mental health. And I wondered where to start.

After ordering a number of lab tests, I discovered Joey had diabetes, high cholesterol, high blood pressure, a gastric ulcer and esophageal erosion, as well as being overweight. He had many risk factors for heart disease and stroke. He drank too much alcohol, smoked, and got very little exercise. He was on income assistance and could barely get by month to month. *Can you imagine living on $600.00 each month? How can you afford to eat nutritious meals, let alone pay bills?* And now, in spite of all this, he had to start making changes, buying and taking medication to control these chronic diseases.

I contacted several local resources to help, including a dietician, who visited weekly, and various community agencies and provincially funded programs. I referred him to any resource I could find, which I felt was applicable to his situation, or I would give him contact numbers so he could make the call himself. I did this not only for the assistance these agencies could provide, but also for the human contact he so craved. Joey enjoyed being around people, and after being isolated for fifteen years, I looked for any reason for him to move toward social interaction.

It was spring, and with a limited work history, I coordinated a referral to a community agency that would help Joey find employment. Due to past injuries to his back, hips and legs, he was limited by a physical impairment, which was aggravated further by his albinism, making him almost blind. By summer, he had stopped smoking, however he still drank, claiming that the beer was his friend. We talked about how the beer – like some friends – can be deceiving and had contributed to his esophageal erosion. Then, out of the blue Joey told me that he didn't care whether he lived or died. At forty-five, he claimed that he had lived for nothing. He had had no friends, no relationship to speak of, his bills were all in the red, yet he still called out for a second chance.

He cried—I cried. We made a contract that he would not harm himself. He was not suicidal, but he was depressed. It was time for medication, to help with this long history of depression. I arranged to see him every two weeks; yet, should he have felt depressed any further, then he would call me, or arrange to go to counselling. The pact was made.

Living and working in a rural fishing town, options are few. The agency where the referral had been made helps with employment, résumé building, and helps toward increasing people's self-esteem, encouraging them to socialize rather than living in isolation.

By late summer, life had already begun to change for the man who had walked into my office only several months previous. Joey had stopped smoking for three months, and had made a decision to stop drinking—"despite losing a friend". He was feeling proud, and as winter arrived, he finally became employed. To some the job might have been considered too menial . . . shoveling up snow for a local church with the added prospect of gardening in the summer; however, for him, it was just what he wanted.

Do you know how expensive it is to eat well and healthy? With a new diagnosis of diabetes, along with high blood pressure and cholesterol, the choice of food, preparation, and portion size were vital. A fixed income of less than $600 per month would not allow him to pay for his rent and living expenses. Joey resorted to eating junk food because "junk is cheaper"; however, despite his reluctance to visit the food bank, he finally agreed to go after much encouragement. Some choices are healthier there—but limited, nevertheless. When he visited my office, he sat on the couch as if he was in the company of a friend, which made him feel like home. He decided to make more changes to his diet, while losing weight and increasing his activity. The physical work would help him to achieve his goal to lose twenty pounds in six months.

My office – small and private – had become a haven for him; and he spoke freely, talking about the past, his childhood, losing his father at a young age and his troubled brother, whom he worries about constantly. We shared possible solutions. Joey was reluctant to seek counselling due to previous unsuccessful encounters, while informing me that I had been his best counsellor. He said that

I had a listening ear and didn't tell him what to do, but instead, helped him to decide on what would be the best way forward.

The weeks and months passed by, and with the New Year came literacy training. He was proud to tell me one day that he could finally read a book, write, and sign his name. He told me how much I had helped him throughout the process. I told him that he had done all the work. And then we hugged. He was so excited, and he had tears in his eyes, overjoyed that he could now read prescriptions and any notes or advice I had given him.

By the following summer a national agency had helped with the cost for new, much needed glasses, and as a result his vision had improved. By the autumn, two years had passed since he had quit smoking—eighteen months since he had stopped drinking. We were very proud! It seemed the second chance he had wished for had arrived: Joey had become happy with his life, he had lost twenty pounds, with goals for further weight loss expected.

Over the next three years, he participated in a daily workshop for those with disabilities. He attended a conference called "A Home of My Own", which demonstrated how individuals with intellectual disabilities could live independently. After the conference, Joey returned to my office with a new goal. He wanted to own a home. He became a member of the local men's service club, helping with a Community Garden Project. He participated in a walk during Disability Week. He became a public speaker at a conference held by the Provincial Association for Community Living, speaking on his personal life and how he overcame obstacles and maintained a positive attitude. He was called their hero. He also volunteered to work at the high school cafeteria while making meal deliveries. In addition, he participated in the Special Olympics at bowling and continued his attendance at any tournaments that were held.

In that same exciting year, Joey became engaged and got married. I was proud to go to his wedding. It was a happy time.

In the fall after his marriage, Joey and his wife accompanied a local government official on a government jet to take part in the fiftieth anniversary of a local disaster, when many years previous a freak storm had claimed the lives of thirty-five men and boys. Among the dead were Joey's father and grandfather, both of whom had perished a month before he was born. This proud man had been chosen to place a cross in memory of his loved ones. It was a sad time for him—but one of closure.

Six years later, Joey remains alcohol and smoke free. He has moved to a new subsidized housing complex with his wife. They attend the centre every day, where he is very active in sports and volunteers at the local food bank. He is an advocate for poverty issues in rural areas, and attends workshops to raise the profile of those living on limited incomes. He was invited to speak with the minister of a government agency about his experiences with work and volunteerism.

One day – not too many years later – someone called in my birthday to a local radio station. Joey came running into the health centre, and said that he didn't have a gift for me; however, he couldn't forget to wish me a happy birthday. This was the best gift of all, and to this day he has never forgotten my birthday.

For the past three years, Joey has worked for two days a week at a local pharmacy, stocking shelves, greeting, and helping out in any way possible. It has been a joy to see him working and had become a valued employee . . .

welcoming customers with a friendly smile, telling jokes, and helping them to find what they want in the store.

Seeing him today, he may not look so different, and thankfully he is still the giggly and happy-go lucky person I have grown to love. He has overcome many obstacles in his life and has never looked back. He is now able to make good eye contact, and with his head held high, he expresses his gratitude. He tells me I was the one who listened and gave him that second chance.

This is barely a snapshot of Joey's life as I know it, but with strong community partnerships, and taking small but workable steps to meet his goals, I feel we have helped him succeed in life and realize his full potential, and I am proud to have been a part of his journey.

I am so proud of my profession. I am proud to be a Nurse Practitioner.

This is the End—Or is It? Palliative Care

Calvin Pelletier NP-PHC, CHPCN(C)

How long do I have to live? is the question asked by almost every patient that I have encountered working in palliative care. The question is complex and often approached with apprehension as well as optimism.

I have had the privilege of providing palliative care to a variety of patients for the past five years. The following stories are renditions of courageous battles I have seen patients wage, and the suffering and fear they endure. The Community Care Accesses Centre (CCAC) Pain and Symptom Management Program provides in-home care for patients of all ages. The program works closely with a multidisciplinary team of nurse practitioners, physicians, registered nurses, personal support workers, occupational therapists, physiotherapists, and social workers. We receive our referrals from the community and primary care facilities. Our program will follow patients from diagnosis to death, and will work closely with the families to keep their loved ones at home. We also utilize the local hospice when symptom management at home is no longer achievable.

The following short accounts are typical of what I encounter in my privileged role working in palliative care.

The Final Days

The house was dark with the faint smell of urine and years of closed windows. The patient was a ninety-eight-year old woman living independently since her husband's death twenty-two years prior. Her diagnosis was frailty associated with advanced age. The reason for my involvement was a bladder infection that cursed her with a fall, and a global functional decline that left her permanently in bed. As so often happens with the elderly, once prolonged periods of bed rest occur opportunistic infections creep in, and she was riddled with various infections. Recurrent chest infections resulted in an irregular heart rate, and then a heart attack. Her final days were made comfortable by a concoction of pain meds and sedatives which I monitored.

During the initial stages of the decline, and being of sound mind, she made a profound statement that is not uncommon among the dying: "I should have died when I was ninety." We discussed the challenges associated with a slow, progressive decline in health and loss of independence. This developed into a wonderful working relationship, and we both learned about our life experiences and challenges with aging.

We have all experienced loss in one form or another, some often more than others. The loss of independence is monumental and eventually the loss of physical life is permanent.

This brave woman passed away peacefully at home, and will again be united with her partner of seventy-six years.

"I Don't Know How to Die"

The house was a shrine to her favourite sport of figure skating. The walls were lined with posters, medals, and other paraphernalia associated with skating. She watched her favourite skaters until the blanket of unconsciousness overtook her. The decline was quick due to a late found liver cancer. There had been various failed attempts of chemotherapy and radiation therapy that bought her some much needed time to get her life in order before her death.

Her responses to my questions were what I had come to expect in such circumstances, except one: "I don't know how to die," she said. We explored this together, with a discussion about life and a strong religious exploration of one's self. As various organs were taken over by the ravenous effects of her cancer, we discussed the physical aspect of dying and the various symptoms she might expect. I adjusted and initiated medications to ensure a balanced level of comfort and consciousness. When the time came, I had the privilege of arriving at her home to be in attendance during her passing. Her skin was the colour of sunflower petals, and an inner peace on her face confirmed that the disease had released her. Her death was private, except for myself, a close friend, and a cat that stayed by her feet until the end.

Baby's First Birthday

The house was stuffed to the brim with kids. Life seemed to go on as usual for this loving family, except for a newly diagnosed inoperable pancreatic cancer. The admiration his kids and his wife had for him was evident in the way they looked at him. In his eyes, fear was present, as he knew my arrival meant he had run out of options, that all treatment had failed. He was worried about managing his pain at home and ensuring he could avoid the emergency department.

We sat on a well-used couch and discussed his limited time. His goal was to make it to his baby's first birthday and give the other kids one unforgettable day with their father. The problem was his advanced pancreatic cancer, eating away at his other organs, causing liver and kidney failure. Realistically, his time frame was only a few days.

We were able to manage his symptoms with diuretics, analgesics, and hope. He had one final baseball game with his family and was able to eat birthday cake with the help of nausea medication. He passed away two days later with his loving and devoted family by his side. I helped the family do some legacy work, and on every birthday they plan to celebrate his life with his favourite foods and activities, and remember him as he was, the bravest father they ever knew. He will be missed to infinity.

The Wedding

The situation was dire that I meet this wonderful man soon, as his only grandson was getting married and he had to make it to the wedding. He had advanced cancer that had failed all treatment except one, hope. The time frame was perhaps one month until his death. We met in the living room he had built himself, with memories of generations on the wall. His family were all present as we developed a comprehensive treatment plan based on comfort measures and a little luck. Antibiotics were utilized for one month to reduce opportunistic infections, diuretics to control edema and morphine liquid to help with pain. In the days leading up to the wedding, we used strong steroids to help improve his energy and appetite. I asked him what his biggest fear was, and he replied he had great concerns of being incontinent at the wedding. We needed to keep his dignity intact, so I arranged for a nurse to arrive the morning of the wedding to insert a catheter and put on a urine leg bag.

Against many odds, he was able to attend his grandson's wedding, and had one more special moment with his family. The combination of determination and some luck gave this wonderful family one final, almost normal day before he died four days later with his family in the living room he built with his own hands.

"Help Me Die"

I walked into the upscale home of a new patient referred from his family doctor. The walls were filled with pictures of exotic travels and certificates of accomplishment. The patient quietly awaited my arrival to discuss the fast approaching end from ALS (amyotrophic lateral sclerosis, also known as Lou Gehrig's disease). Introductions occurred and then the moment arrived. "I want you to put me to sleep, as in euthanize." Unfortunately this was not my first request to end the suffering of someone faster than nature is able to. I changed his focus and suggested that just maybe the healthcare system was not doing enough to manage his symptoms and that we had failed him. In the western world we are ethically and legally not allowed to endorse euthanasia, but perhaps a trip to the Netherlands could be explored. However, given his rapid disease progression and weeks to a few months that remained, this would not be possible.

Solutions were explored and rapid medication titration and aggressive medical management was sought, and the question dissipated, like his control of his muscles. Every week he lost progressively more control, first of large muscle groups and then small ones. Little things like scratching his nose was done with help of loved ones and strangers in the house who helped with all the things we take for granted. The gradual loss of muscles which help with breathing is often the most challenging, for patients and for me, and high doses of medication helped his discomfort. Eventually the request came again at each visit, *please help me die.* Together, we used various trials and concoctions of medications. He died at home from respiratory failure, and continued to ask until the end to be euthanized.

Palliative care is a unique opportunity to help people when they are paradoxically at their most vulnerable and the most optimistic their disease is not going to beat them.

Ontario's First Nurse Practitioner-Led Clinic

Marilyn Butcher NP-PHC

"Never retreat, never explain, never apologize—get the thing done and let them howl"

– Nellie McClung 1916

This is a reflection of my personal experiences during the challenging period of lobbying for and setting up the Sudbury District Nurse Practitioner Clinics (SDNPC), and is not meant to be a research or a historical paper.

"That's it. That is the last letter I will ever write," I said to my husband on July 1, 2006. He handed me a pen and a piece of paper and said, "Write that promise down and sign your name to it." As frustrated as I was, I couldn't quite do that . . .

I had been lobbying all levels of government – municipal, provincial, federal – on issues regarding nurse practitioner practice and employment since I was a student NP in 1995. I wrote letters for my friends, relatives, and acquaintances to use to write their own letters. I had been on the Political Action Committee for the Nurse Practitioners' Association of Ontario (NPAO), written letters that were published in local and provincial newspapers, presented to community groups, municipal councils, and so on it went. The ongoing lobbying had become a central part of my life and I had reached an end point. My family had reached the end point years before!

My NP colleague, Roberta Heale, and I had written separate proposals for NP funding through the recently announced Family Health Team (FHT) initiative in Ontario, and we had both been turned down. In April 2006 we had teamed up again and had written another proposal that had also been turned down. It took some time for us to regroup and recover from yet another disappointment. While attending an NPAO Board meeting, Theresa Agnew, then NPAO President, had encouraged us to challenge the Ministry's decision. Subsequent phone calls to the Ministry of Health and Long Term Care provided no further information or venue to challenge the denial of funding, so writing a letter seemed to be the next step. When Roberta read my first letter, she told me that it was a little too bitter, and it would be best if I tried again. So, one last time to the drawing board. At the same time, we contacted all the NPs in the Sudbury area to get them to co-sign the letter, and as usual, I copied the letter "to the world", not knowing who might respond.

I was an unemployed NP at that time, having quit my previous job a year before. My previous employer had no funding for physician support of the NP positions, and we resorted to running bingo nights to earn money to pay for physician hours so we could have the necessary collaboration when a patient's illness was beyond our scope of practice. Soon, I became disgusted with the premise of encouraging mainly low income people to gamble in order to pay for physician time. When I woke up on that last Thursday – "Bingo Day" – I felt nauseated and frustrated with the ten hours per week I was spending away from patients to earn money for physician support. I felt I had no other choice but to quit, so I became an unemployed NP, after doing a live interview with CBC radio from the Bingo Hall about what was happening. Over the next few months, I contacted various agencies that had NP funding but no NPs, and travelled to a number of locales in southern and northern Ontario to provide locum NP services. Friends in the Sudbury area who did not have a primary health care provider asked me why I couldn't look after them. There were NP positions in a number of places that had been unfilled for years, and I had many unemployed NP colleagues in the Sudbury area. We seemed to be getting nowhere fast.

I was sitting at a clinic in Chapleau, Ontario providing locum services, when my husband called me to tell me that a lady had called about my letter. She went on to say that it was urgent, and that I had to call her back right away. It was Doris Grinspun, Executive Director of the Registered Nurses' Association of Ontario (RNAO). She was incredulous when I told her there were eight unemployed NPs in Sudbury. I assured her it was factual and told her about the numerous proposals Roberta and I had written that had been rejected. Doris was pumped, and it was pretty clear she was going to take action, which was the best news I had heard for a long time. I called Roberta immediately and our planning began: Doris was going to connect with the Minister of Health and Long Term Care, and Roberta and I would lobby both local politicians and NPs. Doris was adamant that we would be successful.

Roberta and I contacted all the NPs in the Sudbury area to encourage them to get involved with the lobbying process. The NPs who were not working as NPs or who had left the area sent in their stories about their lack of ability to work as NPs, all while Sudburians went without access to primary health care. We submitted their stories to the local media, our city council, the Ministry of Health and Long Term Care, pretty much to anyone who would listen. We presented yet again to the City of Greater Sudbury Council and got Council to endorse our proposal, and to lobby the Minister on our behalf. We felt we were finally making some progress.

On October 6, 2006, the Friday of the Thanksgiving weekend, I was happy that my son and his girlfriend were visiting from Toronto, and I was trying to put NP politics on hold for the weekend. Late in the afternoon, the phone rang and it was the Ministry of Health and Long Term Care with an offer – sort of. The two senior bureaucrats told me they had read our proposal and were prepared to fund a two-NP Family Health Team and that for every full time physician we recruited, they would give us one more NP to add to the mix. I was shocked at this offer. It was clear the vision of a Nurse Practitioner Led Clinic was nowhere in the offer; instead, they envisioned the clinic to be a physician recruitment tool. This in a city which was chronically underserved by physicians and whose Family Health Team funded two years prior had yet to get off the ground. As vulnerable as I felt, being unemployed, ethically I needed to challenge their offer. When I reminded them the proposal was for a six-NP clinic at three sites, with the support of a multi-disciplinary team, they replied they were not in the business of finding work for unemployed NPs. The offer would expire on Tuesday October 10 and I was to consult with no one over the weekend regarding this. Despite the fact that I had an apparent job offer, I was incensed.

I immediately contacted Roberta and Doris, and together we decided this offer should be rejected. We decided we needed to intensify our lobbying efforts.

Between Thanksgiving and the annual NPAO Conference in November, there was intense lobbying by all parties involved. Doris worked her magic at the provincial level, and we kept the issue in the forefront in the Sudbury media and with our local municipal council. Another phone call was arranged with the same senior Ministry of Health and Long Term Care bureaucrats. I was curious as to what the outcome would be, and the more paranoid side of my brain thought I should audiotape it, but I didn't. I was shocked to hear them announce they were going to fund the entire proposal as we had written it. Months later, I asked one of the bureaucrats what happened during the month, why they had such a sudden change of heart. He simply said that George Smitherman, (the Minster of Health and Long Term Care at that time), had said to fund the entire proposal. In retrospect, I am unsure as to whether we have ever had another Minister of Health who would have been willing to incur the wrath of the most powerful lobby group in the country – the Ontario Medical Association (OMA) – and give a couple of unknown, grassroots NPs the authority to introduce a new model of care into the Canadian health care system, especially without the input of organized medicine.

This step was a monumental occasion, the significance of which was not lost on Roberta and me. However, we needed to keep our good news confidential until the official announcement at the NPAO conference. The Ministry of Health also needed to inform the Provincial Nursing Secretariat of the coming announcement, and we also advised NPAO of the announcement. At the NPAO conference, it was clear the announcement of the Sudbury NP

Clinic was the Minister's main announcement, and it was met with cheers and loud applause by all. At the end of the conference, a senior nursing official who was speaking to the assembly, turned to me and told me not to mess up because everyone would be watching. So, with that vote of confidence, I left the conference amidst the congratulations of my peers. Colleagues teased us as to how we kept it quiet until the announcement. The media, who accompanied Minister Smitherman, soon gave the announcement wide spread coverage, as did RNAO's communications department.

By the time I arrived home from the conference the next day, the Ontario Medical Association had called my home repeatedly and spoken to my husband, wanting to reach me. I decided my conversations with the OMA should only be via email, so I could track what was said and ensure there were no misunderstandings. In the brief email exchanges that followed, they offered to help us set up the clinic. I advised them we had done this before in other settings, but would be in contact with them if we needed their help. When this tactic failed, they began contacting the Ministry representatives in an attempt to influence the proposal and take a leadership role. Roberta and I advised the Ministry staff that we did not want or need the OMA's assistance.

We were confident that we could be up and running within two months but it quickly became apparent there were many bureaucratic processes that were going to slow us down. During this time, we developed our Business and Operational Plan, chose our first clinic site and did some minor renovations, hired staff, and ordered supplies. Our negotiating with Ministry staff was far from over. During this time, there was a reluctance to fund an Electronic Health Record (EHR) "until we could prove ourselves".

We balked loudly at this, indicating that all the Family Health Teams were getting EHRs without the need to prove themselves. We were also told there would likely only be one NP Clinic, and that we would probably morph into a Family Health Team. Going to the gym after these meetings was helpful.

The Ministry also outlined for us the methods of physician payments in FHTs, all based on rostering patients to a physician only, and the incentive bonus system that remunerated physicians for work that NPs (and other health team members) did. We were to choose one of the FHT methods of physician payment. Intense discussion followed, with us pointing out that physicians would only be involved with a small number of the patients and likely only for brief periods of time. This method of payment was not congruent with the NP Clinic model. In the end, we agreed on the same payment model that physicians in the Underserviced Area Program were receiving for working with NPs, even though it was woefully inadequate and not competitive. We could not stomach rostering patients to a physician in a nurse practitioner clinic.

During this set up period, Roberta and I were working on computers set up in our respective basements. At times I felt like a fraud – who was I to be doing this? We had no organizational support and little in the way of technology to help us. We worked with a business planner who was unfamiliar with working with NPs in leadership roles, so Roberta and I actually completed the majority of the business plan. Two community health care leaders – Gisele Guenard, CEO of Espanola General Hospital who set up one of the first FHTs in Ontario, and France Gelinas, ED of Centre de Santé Communautaire du Grand Sudbury, answered numerous questions without hesitation. We formed our incorporation, set up our Board of Directors, and developed our Board Bylaws with appropriate legal support and a lot of internet searching. These things they just don't teach you in nursing school!

The day that patients would be in the door was fast approaching. Our new Ministry contact, John Roininen, a Sudburian, was a positive support and had a clear understanding of the NP Clinic vision. He advised that some senior Ministry staffers were coming to Sudbury and wanted a tour of the clinic. So, with data cabling hanging from the ceiling and recently delivered medical supplies in the process of being organized, they came with their questions: *What is your promotional plan? How are you going to tell people about the clinic and entice them to come here?* Incredulously, I paused and reminded myself not to let on that I thought this question reflected how out of touch they were. I advised them that Sudbury was a chronically medically underserviced area, that there was a huge unmet need, that the NP role was known in the community due to our PR efforts, and there was a significant level of interest in the opening of our clinic. I was more concerned about our ability to manage the phone lines on opening day. Questions continued: *But, what kind of people would want to see an NP?* My answer was, men, women and children. Followed by, *Well, we know that women like to see NPs.* I couldn't help it any longer. I responded by saying that NPs do more than pap tests, and so I launched into NP 101.

Opening day was a hot and sunny August day. My extended family was at my home for our annual family reunion, and there was a lot of support on the home front. Still, I was on tenterhooks as I drove into Sudbury a couple of hours early to prepare for the event. Would anyone show up? As I came around the corner, I saw people in walkers and wheelchairs heading for the clinic door. It struck me that there was a "sea of white hair" awaiting. Emotions came in fast and furious – angry because these people had obviously been rejected by the medical community in Sudbury, anxious to get these patients in the door to see what we could do to help, and nervous remembering the "everyone is watching" comment. The clinic was located in a mall, with the mall doors opening at 8:30 a.m., and we had targeted opening the clinic doors at 10:00 a.m. so we would have a bit of time to organize last minute items. With crowds at the door, and the hot August sun upon us, we changed our plans and opened immediately, but soon ran out of places for people to sit. I emailed the senior bureaucrat from Toronto and told him that we were overrun with patients at the door.

In the weeks, months and years to come, Sudbury District Nurse Practitioner Clinics drew attention from across the province, country, and beyond our borders. My agreement with the Ministry was that I was a 0.5 NP with a clinical practice, and a 0.5 clinic director responsible for day-to-day operations of the clinic. I soon realized there was a third 0.5 – promoting and advocating for the NP Clinic model throughout the province and country. There was intense media interest and I drew on previous experience in dealing with the media. Years before, I had worked in an HIV/AIDS program in the early years of public awareness of the illness and had to deal with challenging media interviews and public presentations. Nursing organizations and health officials from every province and territory contacted the clinic to find out what we were doing and how we got our funding. We also attended numerous conferences in other provinces, as NPs across the country wanted to hear firsthand how to convince their governments to follow Ontario's footsteps.

Not all media attention was positive, however, and we soon became aware that the Ontario Medical Association had launched a negative campaign about our clinic. They had sent a letter to every Mayor and Town Councillor in the province, encouraging them not to support any NP Clinic initiative in their community. This came after our partnership with the City of Greater Sudbury, which resulted in a long-term lease for our second site in Lively, just outside Sudbury. Many media outlets picked up on the OMA campaign, and without ever contacting the clinic, ran with the story. OMA's talking points were "nurse only"," standalone clinic", "not collaborative", and they questioned our ability to look after patients. This was a deliberate attempt to undermine our NP credentials and the vision of our clinic. Clinic staff who had been working at a fever pitch, going well beyond the call of duty, became upset at this not so veiled attack on their abilities. Patients spoke up and defended this clinic that had not turned them away, and had found so many undiagnosed illnesses in the new patient population.

The Minister's office called to ask how we were going to respond. I advised them we did not have a PR department, and that I had a busy patient load and I needed to focus on patients, but would welcome any efforts on their part. We contacted both RNAO and NPAO about support, and began discussions about a media campaign to raise awareness about the NP role and NP Clinics, but this would be months away. In the meantime, we hired Gisele Guenard, of Visionarease, who helped us develop positive messaging about the clinic. We launched a website and framed a series of positive press releases – NP student graduations, new site opening, etc., and released them on a regular basis. Soon, the Ministry and other health care organizations began to react to OMA's negativity, and over time they wound down their negative campaign. We did not have the time or expertise to engage in a PR war with the OMA.

One day Roberta and I were attending a conference, watching a PowerPoint presentation on NPs, when a slide of the two of us came up on the screen, and the presenter spoke about Sudbury District Nurse Practitioner Clinics. We almost fell out of our chairs laughing and made arrangements with the presenter, Dr. Brian Goldman of CBC radio's "White Coat, Black Art" to come to the clinic to do a show. I was certainly nervous about being "on for the media" for a full work day and exposing the clinic to a potentially negative story. However, the end result was an episode titled *Can Orphan Patients Find a New Home?*, in which Dr. Goldman called our clinic "a game changer", and gave us a huge vote of approval.

Not long afterwards, I was contacted by the producer of a TVOntario show called *The Agenda.* I had never heard of this show, and the producer outlined the plan to have a representative from the OMA, myself, and several other NPs and physicians on the show talking about NP Clinics. I told them I had no interest in being part of a televised debate with the OMA regarding NP Clinics. As it turned out, the OMA representative did not attend the show, and I naively headed out to do the taping at a nearby studio. As I had no PR department to lean on, I tried to frame my message as best I could. Host Steve Paikin's premise was "the doctor is out and the nurse practitioner is in", which was certainly not the message we were trying to send, but colleagues and Ministry officials told me I handled it well.

Conversations and visits by high level politicians were also part of the landscape. As a teenager, my first career aspiration was politics. I thought I had put that aside when I chose nursing. Little did I know there was a career ahead of me that was a meld of the two! Shortly after Mike Harris was elected as Premier of Ontario with his Common Sense Revolution of 1995, he laid off many nurses, comparing them to hula hoops, as a fad that had died away. As part of the political action committee of NPAO at that time, I wrote many letters that capitalized on the hula hoop theme, and received a hula hoop from the organization in appreciation. I kept it for years and finally brought it to the clinic where it now frames our mission, vision and values statements. Whenever any politician or reporter came by the clinic, I would stop in front of the hula hoop while doing the tour and remind them that nurses are politically astute and have long memories. I ensured that when Premier Dalton McGuinty came for his visit in April 2008 he heard the story, and we paused for pictures in front of the hula hoop. The clinic Board of Directors and staff were thrilled when he described the clinic as "the future of health care", along with the announcement of another twenty-five NP led clinics in Ontario based on the Sudbury model.

This story would not be complete without a huge endorsement of the clinic's staff. We brought a group of people who were unknown to each other and invited them to work under the microscope at a frenetic pace. We were the only clinic in town taking new patients, and there was a level of desperation in the community as several hundred patients clamoured to register. Once registered, NPs commonly diagnosed multiple chronic diseases, often in the same patient, as they had not had comprehensive health care for many years. For some patients, the diagnoses came too late, they had been without care for too long. None of our staff had ever worked in a job where patients were so happy to be cared for, yet negative stories were circulating in the media and Ministry scrutiny was intense. It takes a special group of people to rise to that challenge. Kudos to the NPs and administrative staff who weathered those first three years. As time went on, our multi-disciplinary team grew and we are now proud to include registered nurse, registered practical nurse, dietician, pharmacist, and social work services as part of our offerings to patients.

But most of all, kudos to our patients who supported us from Day One. All NPs and RNs have stories of patients they remember throughout their career. I will call my patient Mary, not her real name. Mary was yet another "new intake" on my schedule. She was a seventy-five-year old woman who had been downsized from a previous practice and was accessing walk-in clinics for care, sometimes waiting three or four hours to see a different physician every time. After bringing in hundreds of patients, I was likely not giving my intake process much thought on a daily basis. I invited Mary into the exam room, gave her an abbreviated "NP and SDNPC 101", apologized for focusing in on data entry into our electronic health record, and launched into a health history. Once I had completed "her intake", I provided her with a summary, including what tests I was going to send her for and why, when she should come back for results and a full physical examination, and asked her if she had any other questions. She did. *You mean, I passed?* I was dumbstruck. I had noticed her tremor but had not really understood the anxiety she was under. She had been interviewed by other medical practices and had been rejected. I had never considered not taking her as a patient. From then onwards, my new intake visits always began with, *you are now a patient of Sudbury District Nurse Practitioner Clinics.*

As for the title of this chapter – this was my screen saver for years before the SDNPC story. And so the story continues . . . I left full-time work at SDNPC in June 2010 and continued with my involvement as a Board Director. The clinic has grown to service 5000 patients. However, the clinic's impact reaches far beyond Sudbury's boundaries. I am convinced that Sudbury District Nurse Practitioner Clinics played a key role in demonstrating the value of NP practice, that NPs could run clinics, and this realization affected the government's decisions to expand NP practice and broaden NP scope of practice. This impact can be felt not only in Canada, but in other countries as well when governments are considering their health care options. I consider it a life altering privilege to have been part of such a history-making event and to this day, I enjoy visiting other Nurse Practitioner Led Clinics to experience the depth and breadth of care provided to patients in this model throughout the province.

The Pelvic Diva

Kathryn Flanigan MN, NP-PHC

For most women, pelvic exams or "Pap tests" are a mild discomfort and necessary health check. For Annie, a Pap test re-traumatized her—throwing her back psychologically to when her father raped her. No clinician wants to do an intimate procedure on an emotionally fragile woman, especially if it causes flashbacks. Early in my career as an NP, Annie taught me how to perform a sensitive "woman-first, procedure-second" pelvic exam. At her initial appointment with me, Annie came in shaking and sweaty. She had avoided Pap tests for years but lately she was trying to take more control of her life and health care decisions. Partway through the procedure, Annie "went small" during the exam and dissociated—becoming her six-year-old self. At this point, I stopped the exam. It took several attempts and various techniques to help Annie stay present. Finally, through discussion and trial and error, we were able to complete an entire procedure. I raised the head of the exam table so we could maintain eye contact and to help her stay in the moment. I modulated my tone to be soft and slow, which seemed to soothe her and I also informed her of each step but then also discussed other things, like her newborn niece. Annie, for her part, brought in a picture of her niece to focus on rather than the procedure itself.

It seems so simple now, but NPs and medical students are trained using pelvic models and simulated patients. Also, we are encouraged to use stirrups, foot contraptions that place women, literally and figuratively, on their backs with their legs lifted and separated. I never liked the stirrups—so clinical and cold. The quality of cervical sampling has not been shown to be affected by positioning—with or without stirrups. The semi-sitting position with no-stirrup technique reduces a patient's physical discomfort and sense of vulnerability.

At the Family Health Team where I work, I am a veteran and expert in women's health issues. Female patients can book an appointment with their doctor or an NP. Many women like to have a female provider to perform their pelvic examinations. Furthermore, I have more time for each appointment so we can discuss more than one issue. My focus continues to be client-centred, although I have not often experienced the level of complexity I did with Annie. I have extended my expertise to menopausal concerns: hot flashes, vaginal dryness and urinary incontinence. Physicians routinely refer patients to me for these issues, which is how I met Beth. Beth was sixty-six years old when she was referred to me for urinary incontinence. She had gone through menopause fifteen years prior, and stopped having intercourse with her husband because she found it too painful. She avoided most activities like curling and golfing due to urinary leakage. Sometimes Beth needed to urinate every fifteen minutes. She wore a menstrual pad daily but still did not feel comfortable. She smoked fifteen cigarettes a day for forty-two years. Her cough was also making her leak urine. Beth felt miserable and socially isolated.

I have been trained by pelvic floor physiotherapists to assess and manage urinary incontinence with pelvic floor exercises, commonly referred to as Kegel exercises. Most women do Kegels incorrectly. As an NP, I can also prescribe medication if needed to alleviate the symptoms of overactive bladder and other conditions. With Beth, we started from the top—meaning smoking cessation. She would continue to put pressure on her pelvic floor from chronic coughing. Furthermore, the chemicals in the cigarettes cause bladder irritation. I gave her a bladder diary, a prescription for varenicline (Champix), and a referral for spirometry to assess her lung function. Fortunately, her spirometry showed only mild lung restriction, which was treated with an inhaler to dilate her airway. The smoking cessation medication Champix helped her quit smoking within a few weeks. Furthermore, I treated a previously undiagnosed bladder infection which was aggravating her bladder symptoms. After several visits, Beth was a new woman—she felt confident and motivated to take on more health issues. Switching her to urinary incontinence pads instead of menstrual pads helped prevent flooding and leakage, and Beth was able to comfortably leave the house. I also prescribed a topical estrogen cream to help lower the acidity in the genital area thus lowering the risk of bladder infections.

After a few months, Beth was able to resume some sexual activity with her spouse. It took several visits to modify her lifestyle in order to limit the frequent urinations. Beth's habit of going "just in case" instead of waiting for a signal from her bladder to her brain had caused urinary urgency, also known as overactive bladder. Extending the time between urinations, distracting herself from the first sensation and limiting her caffeine intake all helped her to become the boss of her bladder. It took a few months, but the change in Beth was incredible—she joined a women's curling group and went out more with her family and friends. Her family physician was also astounded at the dramatic change in Beth's outlook and lifestyle. Furthermore, he was impressed with the depth and breadth of the NP role, from smoking cessation to urinary incontinence.

My pelvic diva title is not gender specific, meaning I treat male issues as well. Norm was an active eighty-two-year old who had experienced prostate cancer ten years prior. He was treated with radiation alone and still had his prostate intact. He was now complaining of bladder issues, particularly at night. He would urinate more than five times during the night (once or twice at night for people over fifty-five is normal). I worried about his risk of falls from getting up so frequently at night. A physical examination showed no abnormalities in pelvic muscle tone or prostate size. A completed bladder diary revealed a large cup of coffee prior to bedtime. Furthermore, one of his medications may have contributed to bladder irritation. We worked on behaviour management by stopping his fluid intake after 7 p.m., and decreasing caffeinated and alcoholic beverages. I consulted with his physician about changing Norm's medication to one that would be "bladder friendly". Also, teaching Norm Kegel exercises and other techniques helped improve dribbling after urinating. He was able to decrease his voiding to twice nightly. Norm was surprised and satisfied with the improved sleep and urination.

One of the most positive changes at the Family Health Team is staff actually asking patients if they have urinary issues. I have presented to our staff on urinary incontinence and smoking cessation, highlighting not only the medical issues, but also the NP role. As an NP, I have the time to see patients for 20–30 minutes at each scheduled appointment, as well as the autonomy to decide with the patient a planned course of action. I truly embrace my "Pelvic Diva" reputation and the NP role.

Anesthesia Care and Perioperative Medicine: "I love you, Daddy"

Charlotte McCallum MN, NP-Adult, GDipNPAC

For a four-bed ward room, it was surprisingly quiet. All the curtains had been drawn around each bedside, making it look more like one of those big offices with hundreds of cubicles. Open topped, portable walls were assembled to simulate a pseudo private room, and everyone tried to be as quiet as a mouse hiding from the big bad cat. Having approached the bedside, I called out a "hello", but there was no response. I popped through the break in the curtain, and waved at Mr. Al-Tahar, who plucked at the white cord that hung below his neck. Two ear buds had been sent flying forwards, while his other hand had caught them in mid-air. He then twirled the cord around his fist, finishing the wrap up job in two seconds flat. As a thirty-five-year old computer software designer and tester, he had spent his entire life in front of a screen. His face was pale white—almost a grey-green tinge. His arms were so pale, they were almost translucent. There were stretch marks all over the insides of his upper arms, with skin flaps that looked like turkey wings hanging from his triceps as he lifted his arms. Most people didn't get this condition so young in their lives, and I could see that he had once been a much larger man. Despite being at the height of summer, his skin revealed the lack of sun exposure, like all the typical jokes about a computer geek's lack of tan lines.

After I introduced myself and my purpose related to his care, I asked all the typical questions related to his acute pain after surgery. As I spoke, Mr. Al-Tahar kept his eyes on his laptop, which was propped up on his bedside table. His cell phone chimed and flashed periodically as we spoke, and he would glance at the screen to check who it was before placing it back on his chest, directly over his heart. Evidently he had paid no heed to the warnings printed in the users' information manuals about keeping transmitting devices away from the body to minimize radiation exposure (since the World Health Organization published that this form of radiation "possibly causes cancer"). It is amazing that over 3000 international, scientific research articles have demonstrated ill health effects, especially from long term or over-exposure, yet few North Americans have ever heard about it. Everyone just expects the government to protect them, but there aren't any national precautionary safety guidelines on this continent, so business is expanding as fast as possible in the telecommunications world, before restrictions can be made. Just like tobacco – once everyone is addicted – it can't just be taken away.

As he spoke, I glanced around his environment. His dominant hand had a wrist band issued by the hospital with an electronic tracking device flashing and communicating with the hospital computer system every ten seconds. The nurse stood in the middle of the room with a wireless workstation on wheels as she dispensed medications. She had a wireless, hand held scanning device that she used to laser the medication package label, and then did the same to the wrist band on a neighbouring patient. After she had dispensed the medication to the patient, she returned to the computer and navigated the screen using the wireless mouse. I was in awe that she had been able to perform this without speaking. At the entrance to the room was the antenna transmission device that allowed all these wireless gadgets to silently communicate. The nurse became distracted as her wireless telephone rang. It was someone at the nursing station to tell her a patient needed her assistance. Somehow our modern telecommunications have turned into pseudo mental-telepathy communications. *Whatever happened to human touch and inter-personal skills?*

I continued to scan Mr. Al-Tahar's environment, looking for personal effects. Behind me, I saw some hand drawn stick person pictures on the wall with a scrawled attempt to write "I love you, Daddy" across the top, obviously a heart-filled product of emotion and passion by a very young child. Outside, the sun was framed in blue without a cloud in the sky. The leaves on the trees waved with a slight breeze, revealing their two sides of forest green and a lighter shade of green as they flapped in the gentle wind. I brought Mr. Al-Tahar's attention towards these three images. His eyes diverted from the screen and filled with tears as he described his energetic four-year-old daughter, and how he would like nothing more, than to be able to play with her in the backyard; however, he was bedridden and overwhelmed by intolerable pain.

I found the crack in his virtual world and continued to peel away its impersonal exterior to get to the heart of this human being's life values. Mr. Al-Tahar has been living in pain for most of his daughter's life. Each year the pain had been getting worse, and the doctors were no closer at discovering the cause, yet more and more opioids had been prescribed to deal with the pain. His pain was in the area of his stomach, which was considerably more uncomfortable after he had eaten. But the stomach biopsy only showed a mild gastritis—no ulcers. Mr. Al-Tahar said that ever since he had turned thirty his health had deteriorated. Next, he described an entirely different set of symptoms that were equally as debilitating in his life. He was easily irritated and felt hyper with even the slightest problem at work. He was tired for most of the time, and suffered with headaches after work, a feeling of pressure and constant ringing in his ears that had never gone away. He described a "brain fog" with dizziness, forgetfulness, difficulty finding words and general concentration problems. He explained how he would sometimes wake up at two o'clock in the morning thinking that he heard something, yet not knowing what it was that had woken him. This was exacerbated by the aching in his joints and the twitching of his leg muscles when drifting back into slumber, rendering him tired by the morning when making any attempt to get out of bed, the initial steps causing him extreme pain.

Sometimes his skin was overcome with big red skin blotches, yet according to an allergist, he had no food allergies, just the typical environmental allergies of pollens and grass that stuff up his sinuses at certain times of the year. The pain in his abdomen has eliminated any desire to eat, rendering him with a feeling of nausea. He said that he is now eating healthier, smaller portions of food, only because he is forcing himself to eat something. He has lost one hundred pounds over one year, but the doctors have done every test and still have been unable to discover anything wrong. Over the past five years, he was found to have a low testosterone level, so he and his wife had to go through a fertility clinic, and their daughter was conceived through artificial insemination. After her birth, he developed hypothyroidism and high blood pressure, so he has been on medication ever since. To compound the problem further, it was discovered that he had diabetes, which has proved less of an issue since his weight loss, however, had still caused problems with his blood sugar levels. Over the past year, he has had severe constipation and was hospitalized five times with bowel obstructions. No blood relatives have had the health problems he has suffered.

Once I figured out how to open the flood gates, everything came pouring out. Interestingly, during our conversation, he maintained eye contact and was no longer disrupted by his multiple gadgets. I found the human inside the robotic shell and, once he was given permission to come out, I was blown away with all his life's challenges, emotions and disappointments in western medicine. After twenty-five years of experience, and successfully completing three national specialty certification exams, I have only previously heard bits and pieces of these symptoms, but not all together simultaneously. To have had so many investigations, including exploratory surgery and still be without a definitive cause is incredibly frustrating for such a young family's life, hopes and dreams; precariously, walking the tight rope of an uncertain future. I took a deep breath and wondered where to start with the treatment. I explained to Mr. Al-Tahar, that I would review his electronic chart, his medications and test results, and speak with some specialists and get back to him later that day.

I needed some time to sort out all these symptoms, and to weigh the benefits from the side effects of different medications, to be sure none would add to his multiple problems. Without a diagnosis, it was essential to choose medication that would not add any further complications.

I needed to review his chart to see for myself which tests had ruled out what, but it sounded like a generalized, sustained stress response that had gone wild.

Dr. Hans Selye was an endocrinologist, who lived and worked in Montreal for a period of time. He was the world pioneer in research related to the physiological changes in the body as a result of stress due to illness, injury and emotions. His theories continue to be utilized to further research pathology found in modern day. Going through Mr. Al-Tahar's chart, every medical specialist possible had been involved in his care at some point in time. Every test to explore every diagnosis under the sun had been done. Sure enough, his brain, thyroid, adrenal, and sexual hormones had been altered for some unknown reason—all endocrine related. Somehow he had managed to get a functional MRI of his brain for some research study, which showed pituitary gland, gyrus, hippocampus and other central messaging pathways in his brain had abnormalities. The downside of western medicine, is that every specialist looks at their own specialty, and no one really puts the entire puzzle together. Everyone treats their own specialty as being isolated from the rest of the body. Hence, Mr. Al-Tahar was currently in hospital for an exploratory abdominal surgery trying to find a structural cause for his constipation, pain after eating, and multiple bowel obstructions. This too came up negative on pathology reports.

One thing Mr. Al-Tahar failed to mention was an imaging report that found "osteopenia", a thinning of his bones that could lead to osteoporosis. He also had a series of mammograms done annually over the past four years to watch a lump in his breast, which likely was some thickened breast tissue. Two things typically seen in women, not men, and certainly not commonly seen at the age of thirty-five. His blood work reflected someone who was not getting a good, nutritious diet, and certainly no exercise. For his obese size, he should have had so much more muscle mass, just to carry his weight around alone. However, his blood work reflected a diet poor in protein, and a muscle mass that looked like it belonged to some frail person who weighed around ninety pounds. So, he needed an inter-professional team of therapists and specialists to help him change his lifestyle choices, help address his pain and energy levels, and improve his psychological coping skills in his situation. Unfortunately, not all of that is covered by health insurance plans.

Adding more opioids would only cause more problems with constipation. Since we don't know exactly what would be causing all the different types of pain he has, trial and error would be the only way to tackle such special circumstances. Having high blood pressure that is not well controlled with medications – and considering his body is tolerant to opioids – I decided that adding something that treats blood pressure, boosts the effects of opioids, and treats withdrawal symptoms sounded appropriate. Then, looking at his blood work being low in protein, calcium and magnesium, all reflect poor nutrition. Since some minerals are important in muscle contraction and relaxation, and Mr. Al-Tahar has problems with muscle spasms, replacing his body's normal minerals seemed like a reasonable thing to do.

Interestingly, not only does magnesium relax muscles, but it also increases bowel movements. That's great, because with all those opioids, he had problems with constipation and obstruction. The interesting thing was that Mr. Al-Tahar was not already prescribed a medication to help with regular bowel movements. The other glaring thing was that he did not have around the clock acetaminophen, nor non-steroidal anti-inflammatories, nor a nerve pain medication.

I returned to Mr. Al-Tahar and discussed my proposed medication treatments, along with my reasons. Once I got to the "acetaminophen", Mr. Al-Tahar protested, saying that he was in great pain and that Tylenol wasn't going to work for him. This was a common response from most people who got pain relief from opioids. After I explained how all the medications worked, the side effects they have, and the fact we are not taking away any of the opioids, Mr. Al-Tahar agreed to the plan. He sighed and agreed, saying that I was the expert and that he would give it a go, while apprehensive of the outcome. Most people have been socialized to believe that one pill would do the trick, so trying to sell a juggling act of multiple medications is a foreign and disturbing concept to many people. I was glad Mr. Al-Tahar was willing to try it.

The next day, Mr. Al-Tahar was eating his breakfast. The movie on his lap top was on pause, but his cell phone still chimed frequently. He looked well rested, and almost looked like he had some pink colour in his cheeks. The green-grey colour was gone. Mr. Al-Tahar smiled and said his pain was minimal. He said it was the best night's sleep he had had in years. Looking at the chart, I noticed he hadn't asked for any breakthrough pain killers in the past twelve hours. With admitted disbelief, he couldn't believe how good he felt. We had a talk about some of the free inter-professional services that would be available to access in the community, when he went home. We talked about getting a referral to a chronic pain clinic, which all have long wait times. I described that I would be dictating a summary note to his primary care provider, to make sure this successful combination of medications continued to be prescribed and monitored. I began to explore Mr. Al-Tahar's feelings about alternative therapies. He smiled and shook his head, saying that it was too expensive and hocus-pocus for him. I gave him some therapies that some patients swore by, and encouraged him to at least look them up on the internet to see what they were about. We talked about sitting in the backyard and at least Mr. Al-Tahar could be present while his daughter was playing, so that he felt he was a greater part of her life.

Stress and the immune system work together, to improve or hurt the body. It was such a long winter, that many people had felt the effects of inactivity and a lack of vitamin D from the sunshine. Mr. Al-Tahar and I talked about distraction by interacting with his daughter even if he wasn't physically running around the backyard with her. He could simply sit in the backyard as she played, take his shoes and socks off and enjoy the pleasure of the tactile sensation of the grass between his toes. Being part of summer – especially after such a long time indoors – can change a number of emotions and reduce stress. Tactile stimuli can awaken areas of the brain that are not normally used, adding to distraction from the doom and gloom of pain. Of course, given his translucent skin colour, we also talked about healthy sun exposure and protection for vitamin D production. Spending more time with nature, and face to face interacting time with living beings, reduces stress, it can improve the immune response, and most definitely improves emotions.

I chose to give Mr. Al-Tahar a copy of the note I dictated to his primary care provider. I included the successes we had with the multiple medications we used in hospital. I included the positive side effects and some of the distraction techniques we talked about. I wrote my evaluation that Mr. Al-Tahar's main life value was to be involved with his family. I never heard back from Mr. Al-Tahar, so as far as I know, his treatment in hospital was a huge success. I received accolades from my physician partners at the hospital, for the exceptional work I did in this case. Hopefully my efforts carried through Mr. Al-Tahar's peri-operative experience, to transect the silos of our current health care structure and help him with treatments that should provide him with a good quality of life, no matter what his future health may hold.

The Unlikely Nurse Practitioner

Kathryn Roka NP-PHC

They said I'm in! At the time, I had no idea of what those four little words meant but I was about to find out. I had been accepted into the nurse practitioner program albeit in a rather unorthodox way. It was the Friday of the May long weekend in 2005. I had been sitting with a few friends in my backyard sharing a few laughs and a pitcher of lemonade with the odd splash of Jack Daniel's for good measure. At that time, I had been working for the Peterborough County-City Health Unit as a public health nurse in the Healthy Babies, Healthy Children program for about two years and I was ready for a challenge. I was about to find out that those four words represented my ascent up Mount Everest.

I have a confession to make. Contrary to most who go into caring for others, I never had a calling to be a nurse. In all my years growing up, I never even had so much as an inkling to consider health care as a vocation. I don't particularly like the sight of blood and I have a particular aversion to, shall we say, *suspicious smells.* But that all changed Thanksgiving weekend of 1998: after twelve glorious years in a fast paced legal environment with a near flawless attendance history, I found myself stricken with a virus that robbed me of my strength. I had developed a raging fever that went on for days and lymph nodes in my neck surely the size of walnuts. The worst part was the massive fatigue and nausea that overtook me.

Seemingly unimpressed with my near-death presentation at a walk-in clinic, the doctor suspected that I had a mono.

The kissing disease? I asked in confused disbelief. My knowledge of medical matters was limited at best but I had a vague memory of hearing something about mono from Richie Cunningham and Potsie in the 70s sitcom "Happy Days". *Isn't that what teenagers get?* At the ripe old age of thirty-five, I felt foolish being diagnosed with mono. Surely there was another more plausible and dignified explanation that substantiated my claim that *No one could ever have been as sick as this!*

The walk-in clinic physician went on to explain that I would be off work for at least a month—likely longer. I didn't have time to be sick and I told myself that I would be back to work in a few days. I just needed a day – maybe two on the outside – to get my game back on. But soon I realized she was right. I quickly became an expert on mononucleosis and spent a fair bit of time with my gastroenterologist over the coming months managing an enlarged liver and spleen, not to mention debilitating fatigue that surely would have dropped the Bionic Woman herself. Up until now, I had rarely taken a sick day and avoided visiting my doctor at all costs. For me, going to the doctor was a waste of time and I never gave any thought to the notion of preventative care – but of course, why would I? After all, doctors were for sick people—not me.

Becoming a consumer of health care sent me to a crossroads in my life. In hindsight, I believe getting mono at age thirty-five was the best thing that ever happened to me. I began to think the unthinkable, and how nice it would be for me to help people rather than having to sue people all day long. To make a long story short, I quit my job at the law firm and applied to a nursing program. To say I was taking a leap of faith was an understatement. I was more than a little unsure what the heck I was doing but I truly felt I was supposed to be somewhere else other than Bay Street. I didn't have a calling for nursing, but rather, somehow, nursing was calling me.

Becoming a mature nursing student changed who I was. I was completely caught off guard at my reaction that first time I walked onto a medical-surgical floor in second semester—first year. My new scrubs had that stiff cotton feel with a badge of honour on my sleeve that clearly identified me as a nursing student. It was a little odd as I still felt like a law clerk pretending to be a nursing student—like an imposter. I convinced myself that worst case scenario I was well versed to provide advice if someone had a legal question.

I had little nursing knowledge, skill or judgement to speak of but I felt ten feet tall when I walked the ward corridor. One of my first patients was a man in late stage palliative care. Looking back, I can still see his youthful face thinking he did not look his fifty years. It didn't matter to him that I was just a nursing student. He spoke softly, requiring me to lean in slightly and he let me know he was ready to die. I pulled the chair close to the bedside and I allowed him to lead the conversation. I was acutely aware I was engaging in a special therapeutic moment I had been reading about in my nursing theory textbooks from first term. I became a nurse at that moment.

> Tip: never minimize your ability to make a difference – being present is foundational to the human experience – you can always look up an answer but looking into someone's eyes is what eases human suffering.

As a nursing student, there were many such experiences. There were lots of tears of joy such as those found on the labour and delivery floor and tears of sadness on complex continuing care. I was amazed by the wonderful bond amongst nursing students as we would debrief at the end of each clinical day and recount our experiences with our clinical mentors: good, bad and indifferent. The clinical teachers were phenomenal and would nurture us not unlike a mother hen protects her chicks. And in this safe place to share, there was laughter too.

I remember sharing a clinical pearl of mine. A staunch registered nurse I was tagged with for the day had briskly instructed me we needed to be quick changing the gown and bedding of an elderly gentleman as we were running behind. She handed me a soiled undergarment and pointed to a disposable receptor down the hall. I scurried quickly over to the garbage can to complete my assigned task. As I opened the lid, I made the fatal mistake of taking a deep inspiratory breath. The fumes overtook me and very quickly my breakfast of cheerios was in mouth and threatened to spill onto the clean hospital floor. I had forgotten about my aversion to *suspicious smells!* Terrified that I might be caught throwing up within fifteen minutes of my first clinical experience, I closed my eyes and held my breath. I proceeded to drop the item into the trash and replaced the lid. With great resolve that would have made *Nightingale* herself proud, I swallowed hard forcing my breakfast back down into my stomach, opened my eyes as

I turned and walked back to complete my duties. I must confess a fellow student saw me make my way back down the hallway and called out, asking if I was okay as I looked a little green.

It was during my last year of the nursing program at York University that I first began hearing about nurse practitioners. Fellow classmates spoke of their aspirations to complete the needed years of work experience and then continue into NP education as soon as possible. I admired their calling to greater learning but my goal was to put into action all I had learned in nursing school. I was also mindful that my husband and children had been very supportive of my studies and it was now time to start earning an income and spend time with them. My new second career as a public health nurse at the Peterborough Health Unit was just perfect – straight days and no funky smells! At age forty, I was finished with formal education once and for all and never to return!

> Tip: never say "never" because you will likely prove yourself wrong.

And proven wrong I was. Within a year at the health department, I began to feel I was missing something but I didn't know what. I just didn't feel like a *real nurse* as I went to work in the same clothes and had the same work hours as I did at the law firm. Pen and paper were my clinical tools rather than a stethoscope. I asked myself if I still felt like an imposter. I just didn't know that answer. To try to quell this void I was feeling, I started working causal part-time at Lakeridge Health Corporation on the post-partum floor on weekends. This was fine for a while but I still felt that this was not where I was supposed to be. Something was missing.

And so I bring you back to where we started at the beginning of this chapter. The year was 2005 and I was forty-two years old. Most people at this stage of the game are thinking forward to becoming an empty nester and dreaming of retiring. My friends could tell I was bored and wanted to help.

My friend Deborah asked me if I had ever considered a nurse practitioner program. She and her husband owned their own electrical business so I was impressed she knew about NPs. It was May, well passed the deadline to apply for the upcoming fall semester, not to mention there was a high demand for seats into this program. My knowledge was limited about NP practice but I was open to exploring the possibilities. Perhaps I could get some information and consider applying in a year or two.

My friend found the number for Queen's University and handed me the cordless phone. After being transferred a few times, I finally had the right person on the phone. I let her know why I was calling and strangely she began to ask me very specific questions. After several minutes, she let me know that she had just hung up the phone disqualifying an applicant as they did not meet the entrance criteria. She stated very matter-of-factly that provided everything I had just told her was correct and, provided I could submit all the required documentation by the following week, I could start the primary health care NP program by September. However, she insisted there and then that I tell her whether I was seriously interested.

Oh my goodness! I could feel my eyes widen as I looked at my friends around the table. I really had no idea the magnitude of the life decision I was about to make in literally seconds. In another leap of faith, I replied confidently that I was interested and that I would get her the necessary documentation that she had asked for. After thanking her I set the phone down and looked at my friends with mixed emotions.

"They said I'm in!"

Being a student NP was completely different from my nursing undergraduate studies. The learning was intense, terrifying and exhilarating all at the same time. My preceptors were the most amazing, generous mentors. There were so many experiences of great learning that it would be hard to pick one, however, my last patient as a student was quite memorable. A middle-aged man had presented himself while his new girlfriend sat in the waiting room. At first, he seemed nervous but soon began to speak quickly. He recounted numerous episodes of vicious headaches similar to an "ice-pick plunged into his eye" and it would take him 30–60 minutes to recover while in the fetal position. I asked more and more probing questions intent on getting to the root cause of the headaches. He leaned into me slightly and confided that his massive headaches only occurred during sex. *Oh?* I commented, perplexed by his presentation. I could feel my eyes begin to narrow as I became more suspicious with his next revelation. He went on to tell me that his new girlfriend was very affectionate and he got these episodes four to five times a day. Tugging the corner of his lip as if he wanted to grin he asked me what he should do? To this day, I'm not sure which clinical staff was responsible for my send off to write the NP exam.

> Tip: never take yourself too seriously – laughter is good for the soul.

After successfully sitting the primary health care NP exam in 2008, I worked in several clinics including a Community Health Centre for a brief time. In the fall of 2009, I accepted an innovative NP position with a nine-month pilot project funded by the Central East Local

Health Integration Network, called the Unattached Patient Health Assessment program (UPA Project). The mandate of this project was to provide patients who did not have a regular health care provider with access to primary health care services including physicals, medications, routine screening and diagnostics with referrals to specialists as needed. This was a wonderful experience and I had the opportunity to work with a small team of dedicated professionals. Hundreds of patients who had been previously unattached to primary health care for many years were now getting access, including routine screening, albeit for a brief period. The premise behind this pilot project was that unattached patients deserve the same access to primary health care as those Ontarians linked to a doctor or NP. It was during my time at UPA that I lost that feeling of being an "imposter". One by one, patients would come in to meet me or my physician colleague. We were lucky to have another NP for several months as well. I was struck by patients' stories of not having access to primary health care. They would present themselves to local walk-in clinics or emergency rooms for episodic illnesses but the routine screening, which is a right by virtue of being an Ontarian, was beyond their reach. Throughout my time at UPA, I diagnosed countless patients with considerable chronicity such as diabetes, COPD, hypertension, high cholesterol, and melanoma. When the project completed in May of 2010, hundreds of patients benefitted from the clinical services and the UPA team had the satisfaction of knowing that the quality of many lives had been improved.

I must admit – much to my chagrin – the very first UPA patient got off on a rocky start. I was relieved to know that clinical supplies had been ordered before I arrived. Mr. P. had been previously seen by the registered nurses and was here today for his physical. After meeting with him briefly, I handed him a paper gown with instructions that he should remove all clothing and have the gown open to the back. After ten minutes, I gave a solid knock on the door and entered. My eyes widened as I noticed Mr. P. was sitting in the patient chair with his lower half exposed. To be respectful of his privacy, I turned around and asked him to put the gown on open to the back.

"Sure," he said agreeably. I heard the old chair make a squeaking noise as he stood and the sound of shuffling of the stiff paper gown. After informing me that he had turned the gown to the back, he then told me that it was okay for me to turn around. Relieved, I turned to face him but the situation had become much worse. Mr. P. was now standing before me naked from the waist down. I could feel my face start to turn red in embarrassment as I realized my fatal mistake. Mr. P was wearing a short paper cape used for women undergoing mammograms. A flurry of apologies came out of my mouth. Mr. P. smiled and told me that it was fine, but could he have the other half of the gown, as the old building was a bit drafty.

Another memorable UPA patient was a lovely fifty-year old cognitively delayed lady. The clinic premises were fairly sparse with the bare essentials in terms of medical equipment. In an effort to make the surroundings pleasant for patients, I kept fresh flowers in the exam room. I would be the first to admit I didn't have any flower arranging skills and really felt the pink carnations and white daisies looked just fine shoved into an awkward vase. Miss S., having clearly identified I lacked artistic skills when it came to arranging flowers, asked if she could rearrange my flowers as she waited for me to attend to her yearly physical. I was running a few minutes behind and this would buy me some time. Absent-mindedly, I handed her the paper gown and a pair of scissors. I let her know I would return in ten minutes of so. Shortly thereafter, I rushed into the exam room as I had been delayed helping another patient. As I breezed into the room, I was completely overwhelmed at the beautiful array of flowers cut at different lengths. Miss S. stood there in her paper gown beaming at her work and proceeded to give me a few pointers. It was absolutely beautiful what she had done with the scissors and I thanked her for her kindness. To this day, I keep flowers in my clinic and I try to implement the tips she taught me.

Out of all my patients, I most remember a gentleman a few years older than me – maybe fifty-two years old at the time. He had been without primary care for more than twenty years. He came to visit me one day at the Peterborough Clinic. The UPA project was able to rent a few rooms in the basement of a local building for the last six months of the project. Mr. A. was about 5' 8" and quite underweight. He had been a heavy smoker and drinker for as long as he "could remember". He was very polite and called me "Ma'am". His rich sense of humour was evident when he good-naturedly threatened to submit his dog's stool on the fecal occult blood test kit I was handing him (this is a screening test for colon cancer, where you smear a sample of stool onto a cardboard collection kit). Mr. A.'s hoarse voice caused me concern, and after a CT scan my suspicions were validated: small cell carcinoma. As we sat together, I'm not sure who cried more, him or me. He looked at me and said with a strained laugh, that it was okay. He told me that I had done a bang-up job as he was only supposed to be getting a physical. Mr. A. passed away a few months later. I often think of him and wonder how things could have been different if he had been linked to primary health care earlier.

After leaving the UPA pilot project, I worked at an NP-Led clinic for almost two years. I had the opportunity to work with amazing NPs, including Fran Schmidt, Rebecca Roberts and Julie Lossing. The impressive dedication and leadership they exhibited is a yard-stick by which I measure myself. By focussing on patient access, they went above and beyond the call of duty every day. I am honoured to have worked alongside them. In 2012, I was offered the Lead NP position with a NP-Led clinic in Peterborough. There are twenty-five such clinics in Ontario and it is my honour to be part of this model of care.

These are exciting times for the role of NPs and the one thing we can be sure of is that change is constant, and we will always rise to the challenge.

Rural Nursing Stations: Sink or Swim

Donna Kearney NP-PHC

Nursing stations have been operating in Canada for about one hundred years; usually staffed by a RN and located in the far north, or in First Nations communities. Nursing stations have a mandate to provide care to anyone who comes through the door, regardless if they have a family doctor or not, and no matter how minor or serious their condition is. The nurse is the first point of contact to the healthcare system in these small communities.

The Parry Sound group of six nursing stations are different in that they are each staffed with one NP and are affiliated with the local hospital. They have a proud history of operating in small rural communities surrounding the town of Parry Sound for over forty years. Over this period we were collectively able to demonstrate population growth and stability in these rural communities, something that eludes many other rural communities in Ontario. Rural populations in Ontario have been declining over the years; as people age and require easier access to health care services they tend to re-locate to urban areas. We have found the exact opposite in the communities that have nursing stations in Parry Sound; in fact, the population growth rate in those communities has exceeded that of local urban centres. When rural populations grow, property values are stable, job opportunities improve, and the tourist industry thrives, which is the main economic driver in the Muskoka Parry Sound region.

But more importantly, we have been able to demonstrate improved health for our communities; the elderly stay at home longer and are healthier, the financially challenged have access to care in their home community, and mentally ill and marginalized populations have access to care with the frequency required to monitor and support their needs appropriately. Nursing stations are highly valued anchors in each of these communities.

In 2003, as a newly minted NP, I accepted the position in the community of Rosseau to set up a new nursing station. Prior to that I had been an acute care RN, working in hospital settings for almost twenty years in Intensive Care Unit, Cardiac Step-down Unit, and Oncology units. I had always had the luxury of having a healthcare team around me to support my practice and assist in the development of a plan of care for my patients.

I had never worked in primary care; in fact, I thought primary care would be quite boring compared to the high profile jobs I had previously held. It seemed a suitable form of nursing that would fulfil my current personal needs as a single mother to avoid shift work while I was raising my daughters. I had never worked in a rural community setting where I was the only health care provider and I had certainly never managed a practice before . . . but how hard could it be? . . . at least that is what I thought when I accepted the job . . . boy, was I wrong!

The community of Rosseau is a hamlet in the heart of cottage country. It serves as the summer playground for thousands of cottagers and tourists, but is the permanent home to only a few hundred people, most of whom had never heard of a NP before I arrived. The nursing station proposal was initially written by a group of people in the community who knew the value of having health care to sustain the growth and economy of the village. Cathy Donnelly-Parent, one of the original NPs in Ontario; Alvar Smith, a retired resident and former banker; and Jim Swift, a municipal councillor, wrote and submitted the proposal to the provincial government for funding. Tony Clement, who was the Ontario Minister of Health at the time, funded the proposal as a demonstration project with a whopping budget of $140,000 a year. In other words, "sink or swim over the next three years, then we will talk about more money"! Well, Tony didn't know me then, but he certainly does now!

My office was a sight to behold, a twenty-four-foot construction trailer at the end of a gravel road. I had a sinking feeling in my gut. Was I really making the best career choice or was this something I would live to regret? I had no patients, no secretary, and no job description, not to mention a very challenging budget to work with. I decided at that point to accept the challenge ahead of me and make the Rosseau and Area Nursing Station an invaluable part of the community, and a model for nursing stations across Ontario.

A Community Advisory Committee was formed, made up of local residents, politicians, and business owners. Together we set out to educate the community about NPs: our role, our scope of practice, how we collaborate with physicians and the hospital. I had to demonstrate that an NP could meet most of their health care needs in the community and that they didn't have to give up their doctor in town. I had to earn their trust by being widely accessible and making key community contacts, building relationships with patients, attending and hosting community events. My previous marketing experience with McDonald's Restaurants proved valuable once again, and within two years I had over 1000 patient files – a combination of local residents, seasonal residents, and tourists. At the end of two years, one year ahead of schedule, we successfully negotiated an increased, permanent budget for the nursing station, since we had clearly succeeded in building a sizable and sustainable practice in Rosseau. I hired a part-time receptionist, and implemented an appointment system instead of the previous walk-in system to increase efficiency and security. The community didn't like the change to bookings by appointment, but it was vital to prevent my burnout. We secured daily lab pick-ups, and became a pilot site for the Ontario Telemedicine Network.

It also became evident that we had outgrown the construction trailer and needed to find a new location for the nursing station. I fondly recall a funny story about the trailer – it was not well insulated, and given the types of winters we endured in Rosseau, it became encased in ice each weekend so that every Monday morning I would have to chip ice off the doors with an axe. It became the joke in the community that their NP carried an axe to the office so you'd better not mess with her!

The Community Advisory Committee started a fund raising campaign to have a permanent building erected. By the four-year mark the community had raised the funds, largely through the generous donations of the Carl and Ruth Dare family, to build a state-of-the-art 4000 square foot nursing station and wellness centre for the community. We moved into the new building in 2008 and quickly doubled the number of patient files to over 2000.

Given the dichotomy of the community (complex chronic disease, marginalized populations, frail elderly issues in the permanent population, the episodic nature of the tourist and seasonal population visits), the consistent smattering of urgent and emergent presentations commonly seen in any nursing station setting made this a highly sought after clinical placement opportunity for NP and physician students. I started acting as a preceptor for students routinely, since we now had the space and financial support to purchase the equipment required for the practice. Precepting was my favourite part of the job. I would encourage students to pull together all of the information they had gathered to form an accurate diagnosis and treatment plan. I would watch them nervously complete a task they had never done before and then share the pearls of twenty plus years of nursing experience with them. All of this contributed to my personal and professional growth.

The role of the NP in Ontario was undergoing a huge metamorphosis at the time. It was being embraced by both medical communities and the people of Ontario. The NP scope of practice was expanding to include skills that allowed us to work to our full level of knowledge and skill and become truly autonomous members of the health care team. The pioneering days were behind us and the new era of growth and discovery was upon us. I am proud to have been part of the pioneering efforts in making this great profession come alive for so many generations of NPs that will impact the health care system in the future. NPs have given nurses the voice they needed to gain respect and recognition for our role in the health care system.

The business of running a practice is an entirely different story. Luckily, my pre-nursing career was in marketing and business, so I had an advantage; however, working in a publically funded system only vaguely resembles the corporate world. I am astounded at the amount of self-analysis and practice analysis that comes with running a clinic and with being an NP, the most over-studied profession in Canada. The budget review and data analysis required to satisfy the government that public money was being well spent was also part of the learning curve. In 2010, I decided to do a comprehensive analysis of all six nursing stations operating in the Parry Sound region to determine the impact we have on the local health care system and the rural communities we each serve. The results showed good evidence for further expansion of this model to other rural areas of Ontario. My public and government presentations shifted into high gear and I made it my mission to see this model replicated in other areas of Ontario. Parry Sounds' neighbour to the east, Muskoka, is actively pursuing the funds to develop the nursing station model throughout Muskoka currently.

Rural practice is unique because the people tend to be less eager to seek out health care than their urban counterparts. You see people who are sicker, more complex, and with numerous health risks, often as a result of geographical isolation. I recall a woman who came to my office one day. She was in her early seventies and hadn't sought medical attention for twenty years. She stated she had no trust in the health care system because she had watched her husband die a terrible death from undiagnosed and poorly treated cancer. Based on that experience she had decided that the medical community didn't care anymore. She lived with her son, who insisted that she visit the nursing station. She reported having trouble stirring the batter to make muffins and thought she had shingles on the left side of her chest. She described dressing the weeping wounds by stuffing washcloths in her bra several times a day, but the stiffness in her left arm and her inability to complete her usual activities was becoming more bothersome. I was horrified when I asked her to remove her top and bra and saw fulminating breast cancer – very advanced disease with the breast tissue completely eaten up. I called my collaborative physician – after sending her a digital image of the chest on the Electronic Medical Record – to request immediate hospitalization. A bed was arranged but the patient refused to take it! She stated she had pets and her adult son to look after at home and besides, she didn't want to die in a hospital . . . she just wanted something for the pain so she could live out her final days at home. I believe patients know when they are dying, and I believe they should have the right to accept or refuse medical care on their terms if they are capable of doing so. We changed our approach according to the patient's wishes and supported her at home with pain management, and home care services. She died at home shortly afterward, never having set foot in a medical facility again.

Another woman, who was ninety-four years old, very active and engaged in the community, had a simple hernia repair at the local hospital. She was discharged home a few days later and ripped her incision open while carrying wood into the house to fuel the fire. I was able to not only go to her house daily to pack and dress her wound but also co-ordinated local volunteers to bring wood into the house and help her keep the fire going. Many people in rural areas depend on wood to heat their homes, something hospital staff don't often consider before discharging clients; however, were able to prevent a re-admission and wound infection by providing appropriate care at the community level.

Then there was Theodore; born and raised in Rosseau, never formally educated, but a "salt-of-the-earth" type of person. He would give you the shirt off his back if he thought you needed it or deserved it more than he did. Theodore had been a patient of mine since the early days of the nursing station and during the last three years of his life had a standing weekly visit. Theodore had many life challenges; brain damage sustained from a farming accident in his youth prevented him from being employed so he was very poor. Despite this he lived in his own house that he and his wife built, he hunted his own food until he became too frail, and he grew his own produce in an immense garden that he tended each morning. He often came to the nursing station bearing gifts of venison, fruit or vegetables, or wooden ornaments he had carved.

Theodore suffered from diabetes and heart failure, which progressed more rapidly than one would have expected, but he couldn't afford his medications consistently. Winters were especially difficult because finances were very tight when he had to rely on store bought food, and his heart failure worsened from the work of splitting wood and breathing air from a wood stove throughout a bitterly cold season. One day Theodore came to the nursing station with an ashen complexion, shortness of breath, and chest pain "so severe it would put a horse down". He rode his motorized scooter the two kilometers to the nursing station instead of calling the ambulance. I immediately called the ambulance, applied oxygen, gave him aspirin, assessed his vital signs, did a 12 lead ECG, and started an IV before the ambulance arrived. Theodore was admitted to the ICU with a diagnosis of myocardial infarction. His health status continued to decline over the next three years with several more episodes of chest pain requiring ambulance trips to the hospital, eventually resulting in the insertion of a pacemaker with a built in defibrillator. During the final year of his life I did weekly home visits because he could no longer come to the nursing station for care. Theodore died of multi-system failure; I was with him when he died. Knowing and caring for Theodore was a gift I will forever cherish.

It is not only elderly rural residents who display such stoicism; the young people are equally reluctant to seek health care for what they consider non-life threatening illnesses or injuries. A young woman – mother of five – did not come in for pre-natal care until she was seven months pregnant, and only then because she wanted to make arrangements for her delivery at the local hospital. A young father who cut his leg with a chain saw refused to go to the ER, insisting he would sew it up himself if I didn't do it. And then there was the young mother who felt generally unwell with severe fatigue, but was too busy to seek care until she could no longer walk due to leg paralysis. She was admitted to the ICU with severe progression of Guillain Barré Syndrome and took six months to make a full recovery. Stories like these would make most people cringe. Some may even consider this a failure of the health care system in that these people were not seeking the appropriate level of care when they needed it. But the mere fact that they were coming to the nursing station to seek care at all is an improvement from the past. Lifestyles and values in rural areas are vastly different in so many ways from urban populations and the expectations of the healthcare system are also different.

The rural people of Rosseau, even though they only live a few hours from the metropolis of Toronto, grow up living off the land. They display a hardiness that is uncommonly found in urban centres, and they have learned to be very self-sufficient, sometimes to a fault, as far as their health and wellness is concerned. In order to be a successful health care provider when relating to and caring for rural communities, you must avoid paternalism in favour of partnership, empowerment, and advocacy. In contrast, the summer visitors tend to come in for the tiniest of reasons: slivers, insect bites, even ear wax! Their expectations of the nursing station, and the health care system in general, are very different, often suggesting levels of service should be comparable to those available in urban areas.

Summer brings people to Rosseau from all over the world, the playground of the rich and famous, and cottage country for many people. When people come to the cottage their main objective is to spend as much time relaxing at the dock as possible, to get back in touch with themselves and their family members, and to enjoy a slower pace of living. However, this idealistic view of "life at the cottage", is hampered by insects, partaking in high risk activities such as drinking and boating, and even some of the simple pleasures like walking in the woods can prove to disturb the peace and tranquility of the cottage. At the nursing station we are inundated with summer visitors who suffer the hardships of rural living: infected insect bites, encounters with poison ivy, severe sunburns, skin rashes from water parasites, swimmers ear – all conditions that seasoned rural residents know how to avoid or treat at home.

Then there are the more serious inflictions associated with life at the cottage. I am reminded of a young child who was taking swimming lessons at the village beach and fell on a smashed beer bottle just under the water's edge.

Her entire knee capsule was splayed wide open and blood filled the water instantly. The swim instructor scooped her up and ran with her to the nursing station – a hysterical mother in tow. The child was remarkably calm and co-operative but the mother had to be subdued by the local volunteer firefighters so I could tend to her daughter until the ambulance arrived. In the end the child was transferred by helicopter to Toronto for surgery.

Anaphylactic reactions are another all too common presentation at the nursing station during the summer. Stinging insects are the most common cause, and many people either didn't know they were allergic or they failed to carry their epipen with them. We had one eighteen-year old man with multiple bee stings, who did administer his epipen but had no benefit from the single injection. Already showing signs of respiratory distress, he was brought in to the nursing station by a friend. The ambulance was called immediately, and until they arrived, the next twenty minutes were some of the most stressful moments in my nursing station career. Three additional doses of epinephrine seemed ineffective, Benadryl, oxygen, IV – we were still losing him, he started convulsing! By this time I had the emergency department physician on the line giving me additional orders and support, and I was preparing to perform a cricothyroidotomy (a procedure which involves making an incision into the throat to allow air to enter) with the physician guiding me over the phone, when I heard the sweet sound of sirens approaching. After the paramedics – super heroes in my opinion – whisked him away, I collapsed in the hallway of my nursing station, exhausted, emotional, and scared. I was mentally re-playing everything I had done – *did I miss something, could I have done something differently?* I had never felt so responsible for someone else's life and so alone in making a difference between life and death. I was relieved to learn later that day that he was stable in the ICU, where he remained for a week. He returned to the nursing station after his discharge to thank me for my efforts – that gesture met the world to me!

Luckily, in the summer I usually have an NP student working full time with me. Nursing stations are highly sought after clinical placements because of the high volumes and wide variety of patient presentations we see. We had one summer that was particularly difficult with high acuities and volumes. The ambulance was called almost every week that summer, which was unusual, however, we had patients with burns, chest pains, bleeds, anaphylaxis, lacerations, and fractures. My student, a seasoned emergency room nurse, was an absolute God send!

One day in particular stands out for me. We have four exam rooms in Rosseau, three of them were filled with people requiring stitches and one was occupied by a young woman who was miscarrying her second term pregnancy. The ambulance was en route, the waiting room was full, the people requiring sutures were holding saline compresses on their wounds while patiently waiting for my student and I to be available for them . . . all this, when an eighty-four-year old women was brought in with chest pain and obvious respiratory distress. The patient with the least severe laceration was moved to the waiting room to tend to their bleeding, and my student and I move into high gear to assess and stabilize the patient with chest pain. Starting an IV and oxygen, taking vitals and an ECG, getting a history, medication and allergy list, giving ASA, and trying to get the ambulance to agree to take both patients in one trip instead of sending a second ambulance. The paramedics did a quick assessment of the situation and agreed – against protocol – to take both patients in one ambulance. Once they were safely on their way to the hospital, we settled in to do some sewing!

I remember wondering if the patients sitting in the waiting room thought these situations had no impact on our psyche, and whether they saw this as routine, "all in a day's work" for nurses and NPs. I remember thinking how lucky I was to work in this environment where I have the knowledge and skills to make a difference in the lives of people who enter my nursing station. I feel privileged to work in an environment that offers such variety and the ability to practice to the full scope of NPs practice. I feel lucky to have had the opportunity to inspire and teach NP students in the nursing station, and I feel proud to be a rural practice professional – a specialist in the conditions of rural living.

Rural medicine is indeed a specialty. How many urban health care providers can recognize the bite of a brown recluse spider, the rare and obscure symptoms of Hanta virus, or Lyme disease? How many practitioners consider ground water contamination from road salt when they see several previously stable cardiac patients present with arrhythmias and low levels of serum potassium? Working in a rural practice allows you to care for everyone from pregnancy to death, and everything in between. Rural living brings unique challenges to the health care setting, such as the lack of human services like housing, problems with food security, higher addiction and suicide rates, low incomes and low education. The practitioner is required to work within the capacity of the population to educate, encourage, and assist the people to improve health and wellness. The role of the NP is the perfect blend of nursing and medicine to deliver those services and to collaborate with multiple other disciplines to address the issues of rurality.

Delivering fair, equitable, and appropriate care to rural populations is my career passion. I plan to continue to market the nursing station model and the role of the NP to deliver care in this specialized population through continuing to work with various levels of governments to expand the model to rural areas throughout Ontario, and eventually throughout Canada. Nursing stations are a model that is sustainable and sensitive to the needs of rural populations.

Happenstance

Marnee Wilson MSc, NP-Adult, CDE

I became a nurse by happenstance – a coincidence of life circumstances that turned out to be the most profound thing that ever happened to me. Consequently, I felt inept during my student placements, training alongside others who had been "candy stripers" for years, or beside the diploma-program RN students who seemed miles ahead of me. The academic content made sense to me, but I struggled to understand the essence of nursing as an autonomous profession.

But one day . . . an "aha" moment . . . I began to get a sense of what nursing was meant to be about, at least for me. As a novice nurse, I was working in a coronary care unit and a young man was admitted in the throes of a heart attack, critically ill and needing an urgent pacemaker insertion. Everyone in the room was busy with something: setting up lines, arranging fluoroscopy, prepping the site, taking vitals . . . I happened to be close to his right hand and put my hand over his to reassure him with some human contact and he grabbed my hand. I looked down quickly and his eyes locked on mine – he said nothing.

There were no words. His terror was clear. I felt as though I could see through to his soul. I stopped what I was doing and spoke quietly in his ear, explaining what was happening and why. After a few minutes, his breathing settled a bit, the fear abated in his eyes and his death grip on my hand loosened. And at that moment it became clear to me what nursing was. I understood that this connection – the connection between nurse and patient – was a unique and precious privilege.

Another key event profoundly affected my understanding of the power of nursing: during a morning assessment of a patient I had been caring for, I detected a new heart murmur and subtle cognitive changes in a lady who had suffered a heart attack. I could not recall hearing the murmur on the previous day, nor had the attending physician noted it in his earlier note. I called him to discuss this finding and, after listening to my concerns, we arranged for an echocardiogram that confirmed a new defect. The lady was expedited for emergent surgical repair and survived. This was the first time I truly understood the responsibility of nurses to not just "go through the motions" of assessments. It had become clear to me that what nurses do matters a great deal and could make a real difference if it was done well.

These two experiences changed me fundamentally. I knew that I wanted to have more in my armamentarium to capitalize on the relational experience with the patient to make the experience of illness less severe and traumatic—and help patients be or get well. I needed to have access to a broader scope of both practice and greater power to influence the system and mobilize the entire team to do so. To do this I required further skills – clinical skills. At the time the role of the NP in hospitals did not exist – but I knew there was a fantastic opportunity for nurses to be advanced clinicians at the bedside – not primarily as administrators or researchers or clinical educators, but *fundamentally* as advanced clinicians.

One of the first hospital-based NP roles to develop was in surgical settings, where the ward care often suffered because physicians were often in the operating room. The role initially began as an extension of the physician, but over the years (and particularly influenced by the legislative changes in Ontario which occurred from 2007–2011), evolved into a distinct and autonomous role that leads the care of patients and works collaboratively *with,* but is not directed *by,* physicians.

The NP role in hospital-based, acute care settings is grounded in the unique patient-NP relationship, and uses advanced clinical reasoning and diagnostic skills together with the autonomous NP scope of practice to improve the quality of the patient experience. The goals of NP care in these types of settings are focused on treating the presenting illness while preventing nosocomial (hospital-acquired) complications, identifying and treating them expeditiously; managing pain and chronic co-morbid illnesses, collaborating with inter-professional team members, and managing complex care in a way that uses resources in an efficient and effective manner. NPs in acute care provide care to some patients with relatively uncomplicated acute care issues, but also to many patients with very complex clinical situations that require considerable involvement and energy. The following vignette is one example of an experience with a patient and is meant to illustrate the NP role in an acute care, hospital based setting.

Jason had been admitted to the hospital for elective spinal surgery. On the day following that surgery, he developed chest pain, suffered a cardiac arrest and underwent emergent cardiac surgery. He was severely delirious after surgery and spent many days in intensive care. I met him and his family when he left the ICU, and was struck at the time by the strength of the family who had already been through an unexpected ordeal. Jason's wife Rose and their children were stunned at the severity of his delirium: Jason was the CEO of a large company and the one to whom everyone went for advice and guidance and he did not recognize them or make any sense at all. I spent a great deal of time with them that day, listening to their description of Jason, letting them relate their experience so far, and discuss the plan of care from this moment.

Every morning I examined Jason before Rose came in and he recognized me, but this was often the only moment of lucidity in the day. This became a symbol of hope for the family who weren't there at the time, but wanted an account of the morning visit when they visited in the afternoon. Jason failed to make any real progress despite our best efforts and I undertook another full delirium work up. There were no clinical signs that pointed me in any direction; however, he continued to worsen to the extent that I suspected sepsis (a whole body infection carried by the bloodstream) and began aggressive supportive measures. He was eventually sent back to the ICU where he required full support including mechanical ventilation, dialysis, and blood pressure support. A source of infection was found several days later and Jason underwent urgent bowel resection and an ileostomy for an ischemic bowel. He was transferred back up to the ward several weeks later, with a new ileostomy, on dialysis, yet still delirious. On the ward, he had more problems, including several gastric bleeds, recurrent urinary tract infections and tenuous fluid and electrolyte status.

Rose and I became partners in his care, along with the inter-professional team. Rose was an extraordinarily intuitive woman with incredible compassion and a keen eye for noting subtle changes in her husband's status. She held a unique view of the hospital system and its strengths and weaknesses, and her thoughtful questions provided valuable feedback on the way the unit and staff functioned.

Slowly, Jason began to improve and had more frequent moments of lucidity . . . and gradually these moments became hours. His condition had deteriorated significantly because of his inability and unwillingness to become mobile. One day, during a period of clarity of mind, he decided he wanted to walk with the physiotherapist – a miracle! His physical endurance had deteriorated significantly because of his inability to mobilize, and he had not walked in months. Rose was not there to witness it but we caught the moment with a camera (with Jason's consent, of course) and shared it with her when she came in.

As he became more lucid, he began to chafe at being in the hospital and begged his wife to go home, although he was still delirious some of the time and his gait and balance were unsafe. Rose began to speak about taking him home as he was, but I felt that he was not ready and that she would not be able to manage his requirement for constant supervision and assistance despite the home care we had requested. Rose was convinced he would improve in familiar surroundings and surrounded by family, and was determined to try and take him home. Somewhat reluctantly, we worked together to prepare them as best we could; she had to learn how to manage the ileostomy, monitor and maintain his fluid balance, and how to cope with his persistent intermittent disorientation. Working with the Occupational and Physiotherapists and community services, we arranged as much home support as possible and sent them home – still not happy about it, but respecting the courageous and loyal decision Rose and the family had made.

As we had feared, things did not go well at home. Jason did not recognize his surroundings and worsened to the extent that he became aggressive and required admission to the small local hospital. The local hospital concluded that Jason also had severe dementia and recommended long-term care, but Rose disagreed and had him assessed elsewhere. Reassured by the second opinion that this was not dementia, she took Jason home again and this time he thrived. Jason is now completely free of delirium and back to work at the company he founded.

As the NP responsible for the care of this patient and family, I felt that my role was to carefully assess and manage Jason's complex day-to-day issues and design the overall plan of care, but perhaps more importantly to help Jason and Rose navigate this devastating period in their lives. From the family's perspective, I was the "glue" that held things together. I was humbled and honoured to witness the devotion of Rose and Jason's children and to help them integrate this experience into their lives and support their roles in helping their husband and father to heal.

The foundation of NP work is embedded in the responsibility of connecting with patients at vulnerable points in their lives and leveraging the advanced clinical skills and scope of NP practice to influence the patient experience of illness and wellness. What we do with this privilege is up to us.

Paving the Care Path to Excellence in Geriatric Health: The Senior Tsunami

Michelle Acorn DNP, NP PHC/
Adult, ENC(C), GNC(C)

The opportunity to focus on senior care is greater today than ever before. Targeting the quality agenda in an effort to respect our valued citizens and veterans who have given so much to us and have years of wisdom to spread to us must not go unnoticed. A serious lack of geriatric curriculum is evident in both nursing and medical schools. Geriatrician shortages became the driving force for my nursing colleagues to excel.

Geriatric Emergency Nurses (GEMs) are now a tremendous asset positioned in most emergency departments (ED). They are advanced practice nurses, either functioning as a Clinical Nurse Specialist (CNS) or Nurse Practitioner (NP). Their mandate is to identify and link with seniors at risk for hospital admission to address many of the geriatric syndromes (falls, polypharmacy, depression, delirium, drugs, and frailty). Delirium (acute confusion) can be life threatening for seniors if not recognized and treated by identifying and reversing the cause. As well, many seniors are discharged from hospital in delirium.

GEMs also support staff capacity for better senior care and link seniors with community resources to keep people supported in their homes (PSW support, nursing, mental health support, Meals on Wheels, home safety reviews, physiotherapy, occupational therapy) or liaise with long-term care residents and families to prevent ER visits or expedite discharges to their homes. Prior to my role in geriatrics, when a senior presented with a fall resulting in a laceration or fracture, as the NP in the emergency department I would suture their wound, set their fractures by casting, or consult with the orthopedic surgeon for surgery to fix their broken hip. The focus at that time was on episodic focused care with a goal for discharge, as opposed to a comprehensive geriatric assessment approach to reduce risk, optimize chronic disease management, and support health.

The senior who falls will now receive senior friendly care. Vital signs assessment would look for blood pressure lowering changes causing them to get dizzy and fall. Medications would be reconciled and reviewed looking at prescriptions, over the counter agents, and alcohol use for potentially fatal drug reactions. A health literacy lens would ensure a senior's knowledge and understanding of why they were taking their meds, accuracy of administration, system support such as blister packing for compliance, and reducing medication burden by identifying and removing potentially inappropriate medications. Seniors taking Gravol and Ativan for insomnia, for example, would be educated regarding the increased risk to their brain, causing sedation, falls risk, confusions and dependence concerns.

One of my most rewarding experiences was with the Specialized Assessment of the Frail Elderly (SAFE) clinic. The greatest predictor of a fall is a previous fall. Strikingly, once every five seconds in Canada a senior presents to the ED due to injuries related to a fall. Thirty to fifty percent of seniors who fracture their hip die within one year. Many of the seniors who survive have reduced quality of life from reduced immobility. Others develop a fear of falling and lack confidence in their walking mobility resulting in social isolation, and deconditioning. This opportunity with the SAFE clinic presented as a result of a hospital fire that resulted in its closure for over four years. We were the first hospital to experience a devastating fire and successfully evacuated almost a hundred frail seniors. These poor seniors were uprooted and displaced to local venues who helped accommodate us. Many had dementia and became acutely confused. The strength and resiliency of the patients, families and staff demonstrated true heroic qualities. The fire was an adrenaline rush to get people to safety. Counter this with the need for calm, professional and emotional intelligence. I vividly recall one of our seniors bragging about the wonderful therapeutic activities that we have with firefighters!

The SAFE Clinic has now evolved into Geriatric Assessment and Intervention Networks (GAIN), an interprofessional team, which includes physiotherapy, occupational therapy, pharmacy, social work, home care, and geriatrician support. This model of senior care was developed in an effort to keep them supported in their homes and reduce emergency visits. Four GAIN clinics with community outreach now successfully exist to meet senior health needs.

My next senior journey took me along the path to true inter-professional care. A collaborative NP model innovated the health care landscape and evolved into the first NP-Led hospital in Whitby, Ontario, and in the world to our knowledge. The patient population focused on seniors who required geriatric rehabilitation, complex care, and alternative level of care while waiting for long-term care beds. Seniors are transferred from hospital to this post-acute specialty service once they have been stabilized. The specialty service utilized the NP as Most Responsible Provider (MRP), traditionally a role held by physicians. Many of the patients admitted to the unit were frail and deconditioned due to prolonged hospitalization, and were experiencing acute confusion (delirium) from the insults of surgery, and multiple medications. The most rewarding professional journey by far was the shift to forge this new model of hospital NP care. It has been almost ten years and remarkable to see the health care landscape paradigm shift. This was a significant shift from the traditional physician led model of care from admission to discharge. Due to recent changes in legislation in Ontario, NPs are able to admit, treat and discharge inpatients from hospital. NPs are disruptive innovators who challenge the status quo. Our team was the first in Ontario and Canada to implement the full model of care with the NP as MRP. This was the driver of my doctoral research. The results were very positive. Patients, families and staff were satisfied with the quality and safe care provided by the NP as the MRP from admission until discharge.

Patient stories are in the hundreds. Mr. Reed was transferred to our unit after an admission related to a urinary tract infection, resolving delirium (acute confusion) and progressive dementia (memory loss). He was awaiting admission into a long-term care facility and required a secured locked unit due to physical and verbal aggression and elopement risk (leaving). Upon the first early days on our unit our team successfully utilized gentle persuasion techniques for dementia, such as redirection and distraction. He had over fifteen medications prescribed. I initiated a slow taper of antipsychotic medications (potent mental health drugs) in an effort to reduce his risk for stroke, heart attack and falls. With this medication tapering (slow reduction/withdrawal of medications) his physical restraints and urinary catheter were stopped to align with best practice guidelines and patient respect and dignity. Mr. Reed became mobile as a result of these changes and his aggressive behaviours also stopped. He had a kind and gentle disposition, showing affection to other patients and staff on the unit. He was able to be discharged to a retirement home instead of a long-term care home, and was able to remain independent, yet supported for any health needs such as meal and medication adherence. His daughter was overwhelmed with gratitude and appreciation!

Many patients are admitted to hospital to await long-term care placement due to dementia. The progressive nature of dementia as it advances from mild, then moderate through advanced disease is under-recognized and often not addressed in terms of understanding for end of life care. Palliative (end of life) considerations need to be realized and discussed not just for cancer, but other complex chronic diseases such as advanced dementia, chronic obstructive pulmonary disease (lung disease) and heart disease. During their terminal disease phase, patients have progressive weight loss, reduced appetite, reduced mobility (stay in bed more), and increased sleep needs. Many have dysphagia (difficulty swallowing) and complications from aspiration pneumonia (lung infections). Crucial conversations should explore options for Power of Attorney for health, residence and finances when the patient is unable to make these decisions for themselves. Prior patient preferences and wishes need to be shared in advance with loved ones to aid in ensuring decision making is respected and upheld. Many people choose a "do not attempt resuscitation" (DNAR) option, meaning no cardiopulmonary resuscitation (CPR), no intubation (breathing tube) or ventilators (lung machine), making way for a natural death.

Many elect to forgo artificial hydration (intravenous) and artificial nutrition (feeding tubes) and dialysis (kidney machine), not wanting to sustain their own lives without quality, especially when their unfortunate fate is not being able to return to home and being totally dependent upon others for their care needs. Many patients appreciate the NP education to understand their story and prognosis for future health and illness. A good death, pain free with supportive family and friends is the goal that NPs can advocate and support.

One of my most rewarding patient experiences was to relocate a veteran to spend his last days with his daughter in western Canada. It was a true demonstration of team collaboration that was exhilarating. The Social Worker on the unit worked with the family to search out various travel opportunities, from accessible RVs to aero-medical and ground transportation, balanced with what I could do to medically stabilize him for the trip. In the end we were able to utilize a commercial flight with medical supports. We were all in adventure mode, including our veteran who was more than up for the challenge. He arrived safely and his family was in tears with gratitude.

Sometimes it is not only the patients we assist, but it is also the families. In one case, we had a patient whose husband had a dream to be with his family on the east coast of Canada, as he had no family here and limited friendships. He had been laid off from work and often would be found wondering the halls of the hospital seeking social interaction from the staff, as his wife was no longer able to carry a conversation or acknowledge his presence. He worked with our team in preparing and planning for her transport to the east coast with him when she died. He had no family and no friends as he sat with her crying. We were his professional family in those low moments as we took turns sitting with him until he was ready to let her go and move forward with his dream to return home. He made his move and we continue to receive calls from him from the east coast sharing with us his new life, his supports, and invitations for visits. Each call is never without appreciation, gratefulness, and an expression that our team has healing hands, even if a life ends.

One of the most interesting projects I have been honoured to support is the "Life Gifts from Our Oldest Population at Lakeridge Health Whitby" project. As staff we are often exposed to what our elders in the hospital truly feel about themselves, and most had been expressing a lack of value. They felt they were a burden to their families and that they had nothing to offer society, and felt they had a lack of purpose. What could they possibly give when they needed someone to take them to the washroom and they live in a hospital? As staff we were also exposed to those precious moments of wisdom, such as these words from an eighty-six-year young patient: "It doesn't matter what colour your eyes are. It's what you see from them." And then, a magical idea was born to collect the quotes of our patients and to mount their quotes via a car decal onto a donated 1992 Nissan Sentra with 430,000 kilometres on it. This car would be driven around the community showcasing that our elderly do have a purpose—a gift to give. It does not matter where you live, what your health is like, or what you need help with, you still have a purpose and that is always in the power of your words. It was a unique project that created "inspiration" for our patients, and staff and a life gift to our community.

Sometimes our own systems can be a barrier to care, as was the case with a young man who came to our unit without complete mental health treatment due to his refusal of treatment. Our team had an amazing rapport with him and his family, as he had many similar interests as our staff due to similar ages. His outgoing personality and humorous disposition began to get lost in his mental illness, as he continued to refuse the treatment he required. Despite the efforts of counselling and the use of community based mental health agencies he spiraled into a psychotic state and stopped eating and drinking. He truly needed emergency psychiatric intervention. His family were struggling with his wishes to die and wanted to honour his wish, yet struggled with the mistrust they had developed with previous mental health services. In this moment, rapport was critical. The family blindly trusted us as we eventually transferred him for the appropriate treatment. He returned to our unit a different person and the family felt "he was back". As a result, we now have contracted services with a local mental health hospital for on-site psychiatry consultations.

My wish is to transform health care through advanced practice nursing clinically at the bedside, sharing knowledge through research and education and leading professional change. Knowledge is power, it leverages capacity and networking opportunities. As Johann Wolfgang von Goethe said: "Knowing is not enough, we must apply. Willing is not enough, we must do." If your actions inspire others to dream more, learn more, do more and become more, you are a leader.

Despair and Hope

Natasha Prodan-Bhalla MN/NP (A), DNP (c)

Susan sat across from me staring at the floor. She was in a wheelchair that had a dirty cushion and mud on the wheels. Her wheelchair was banged up from various incidents she had had with it, as being an alcoholic, she had bumped into things when she had been drinking. As well as her alcoholism, she was very loud; she suffers from obesity, diabetes, chronic obstructive pulmonary disease (COPD) from years of smoking, and high cholesterol. Susan has not taken any form of medication; her life has been chaotic and therefore has not lent itself to any consistent use. Susan's husband is a drug dealer and has an addiction to cocaine, while she too has been a drug addict, however, she has been clean for over ten years. She has three sisters, yet their contact with each other has been inconsistent over the years. Susan sees me at a resource centre in the inner city, where a group of NPs run a primary care clinic during the week. We have many patients like Susan. We attempt to provide primary *health* care and not just episodic care, but this tends to elude us more often than not. Susan sees me regularly—sometimes just for support and to check in with me. She sees no other health care provider outside of the NP clinic.

When I first met Susan, I was fairly new to the harshness of the downtown eastside. She has taught me a lot in terms of resilience and what it takes to survive day to day. She first came to see me for a problem she had with fainting. She would get out of the wheelchair to move around her apartment and would often fall, however, when I asked her how she fell, she was unable to give me a straight answer. She had little recollection of what precipitated the fall, and lacked knowledge of any medical history that may be contributing to the problem. She had been in an out of a few walk-in clinics in the area over the last few years and had also been in the care of another primary care clinic in the area, but she was not happy with her treatment there so had been floating from clinic to clinic over the last few years with no consistent care. After ruling out the emergent issues such as a transient ischemic attack (TIA, or "mini stroke"), stroke and arrhythmia (irregular heartbeat), we settled on a few initial baseline blood tests to see if there was anything metabolic going on.

Susan didn't get the testing done and I didn't see her for a few months after that. We had also arranged that I would try and get her old records to understand her medical history a bit better, and we agreed that this might help me understand what was going on with her so I could help her more effectively. Her previous clinic did send me some old test results, however, nothing recent and there was no history of fainting. At Susan's next appointment, she said the fainting had subsided and she thought it may have been due to low blood sugar. However, she hadn't tested it and she couldn't remember the last time her hemoglobin A1C was done (a blood test which provides a measure of average blood sugar readings over the past three months), but she was sure this was all it had been. She was not interested in any more tests, referrals or medications.

Susan is noted for being extremely difficult to connect with and care for. Her attitude is gruff and she has neglected many follow-throughs on any management plans that we have developed together. She gets upset regularly and often cries in the clinic. Yet, she comes for her appointments and clearly relies on us for ongoing support. The resource centre has provided a family for her and a safe place to spend her time away from her abusive husband. She has spent much of her time on the computer, researching issues that have been causing her concern, such as the issue of homelessness.

We often see Susan for forms that need to be filled out: forms for her wheelchair, a special diet, Occupational Therapy (OT) and Physical Therapy (PT) assessments, forms for bus passes and numerous other accommodations she requires. I had her assessed by OT a few years ago and according to their report, they saw no reason why she needed to be in a wheelchair and encouraged us to stop any further application for wheelchair assistance. However, she insists that she is "weak" all the time and "passes out" regularly, that she has never been steady on her feet and has had some kind of stroke in the past that is undocumented. Susan lives upstairs from the clinic in a single room occupancy building. These buildings are infamous in the downtown eastside where she lives, and they are often rampant with bedbugs, cockroaches and rats. I have written to her landlord requesting that an effective spray be used to tackle bedbugs and eradicate any other health hazard that she may be experiencing. I always find it hysterical to write these letters, as isn't this obvious enough? Yet, I find myself writing them time and time again.

The next time Susan came in to see me it had been raining and the clinic had the scent of a wet locker room. She had wheeled in to the clinic and having heard from a friend that the rules for housing were about to change, which would present her with the opportunity for better housing, she had been in good spirits. Although this never came to fruition, it had still proven to be a good day for Susan—days that were infrequent and therefore she would require my support wherever possible.

She had told me a joke and spoken of her excitement for that particular evening when she was expecting a visit from a friend. During her clinical encounter, she had disclosed that her husband had hit her the previous night when she had been asleep, an assault that had come out of the blue, however, one that had caused her to fall out of the bed. She didn't know why or how it had happened, but she was bruised on the left side of her body.

Having asked her if she had fallen on her head or had hurt herself anywhere else, she had said that she thought she was okay and so didn't want to discuss it any further, so as not to ruin her day. I decided to follow her lead and so we moved on.

One time Susan came to see me for help with a letter she was writing to get better funding for improved housing. She had been waiting for years for a room of her own so she could leave her abusive husband. On this particular visit, it was sweltering outside and the fan was whirling by our feet. We could hear women outside the clinic room talking about the previous evening out around town, and that one of them had "got into a bar fight and got hurt", yet remained unconvinced at that time that there was any need to come to the clinic. She felt it was just bruises and they would heal.

Susan proceeded to tell me about the letter and her wish to frame it in such a way that her health was being affected by her poor housing. A friend had told her that this might work better than just requesting a better place to live. The letter was dirty and crumpled, and there was a strong, unpleasant odour coming from Susan. I wondered when had been the last time she had taken a bath or shower. I understood how difficult the situation was for her and worsened by the fact that she also struggled with incontinence. She would not let anyone into her apartment, so getting her help was not an option. I asked her how things were going with her husband. Was she getting closer to leaving? What was going on in terms of her health? She felt her diabetes wasn't very good but was reluctant to go for any testing. She was not open to discussing why, she just didn't feel like it. I suspected she was drinking again, but she denied this.

She had remained sullen and quiet throughout our encounter, which made me wonder why she had presented herself with the letter at this time. I knew her well enough to be able to see there was something else bothering her but she was not ready to disclose what it was. I asked about her fainting, at which point she had started to cry, telling me that overall she just wasn't doing well. I wondered about depression but we had gone down this road before. She was reluctant to get counselling or take any medications for depression. She had been on an antidepressant in the past, which she admitted had been helpful, but she stopped taking it anyway.

There was another occasion when Susan came to see me, determined that she was going to leave her husband once and for all. Susan had taught me that loving an abusive partner is possible, however, she agreed that a safety plan was in order, which was something that we continued to work on. She has someone to call if she needs to – even in the middle of the night – and I've given her numerous crisis line numbers. She sleeps on the side of the bed closest to the door and has essentials packed; still, other than her monthly disability allowance, she has no money, and therefore has had no need to form a financial plan. Any funds from her disability has paid for the rent, the rest has gone toward her husband's drug addiction, which has undoubtedly led to considerable risk for her as strangers sometimes come to her apartment.

She often tried to leave, but the wheelchair made it difficult, although she has admitted that she can get around her apartment without it if she needs to. She has tried to keep whatever money she has away from her husband, to save a little each month in the event that she is able to move out on her own. Susan felt that her husband's money helped to pay for food, but doubted that he had enough intelligence or knowhow on how he would go about following her, so she made plans to move as soon as possible.

We had discussed this on and off over the years, but she seemed more determined that day, more insistent that she was going to follow-through, more insistent that she had the strength to do this. I asked her where she was going to go, and she replied that she would go to a local women's shelter. However, she requested if she would be able to leave some of her belongings at the clinic from time to time in case anything might be stolen. I said I would try to find out from the staff if it would be possible to do so, yet I knew that they would be reluctant to do so, fearful that they might be setting precedents.

Susan was very well thought of by all the staff and, after much discussion, it was agreed that she would be allowed to leave some of her belongings at the clinic on a temporary basis. There was, however, a concern that some of her belongings could contain bedbugs, therefore we decided to use double garbage bags to ensure we eliminated any risk of infestation.

A month went by and I didn't hear anything about Susan. I kept asking the staff if she had dropped off any belongings at the clinic, but neither one of them had heard from her. I was really worried about her safety. I was concerned her husband had found out that she was planning to leave him, and he had hurt her badly. I called her rooming house numerous times but she wasn't there. I left messages and she didn't return them.

Then one day, I saw her at the clinic, sitting in front of the computer. Susan was elated to see me. She raised her arms and exclaimed: "I did it!" Her few belongings were at the clinic and she had left her husband as planned. She felt so relieved, tears started streaming down her face. She was so grateful for our help and felt so strong and proud of herself for having carried out her plan. Her husband hadn't tried to find her and seemed to accept that she wanted to leave. I was so relieved.

Susan was a perfect example of the patients I have seen in my practice. *Do I wish I could do more from a health perspective?* Yes, of course. Susan had diabetes that wasn't being monitored or treated; she had untreated high cholesterol, and quite likely liver damage from her alcohol use. She was not doing regular physical therapy to get out of her wheelchair, and she was not keeping the appointments that I was constantly arranging with the counsellors. However, we were there for her when she needed it—on her terms, not on ours—and we did the best we could under the circumstances.

One step at a time . . .

Being Brave and Reaching Out

Lorine Scott MN, NP (F)

My inner city has a vibrant aura, and it is a clash of cultures and ethnic backgrounds. It is typical of many inner city neighbourhoods, both picturesque and run-down, with old homes and dilapidated apartment buildings, some newly renovated but most in disrepair; there are parks and community centres, some are safe and some are not. There is poverty everywhere amid upper- middle-class folks. And there is a school, because of course children live in this community. It is here my story begins.

It was a typical day in my inner city outreach practice. It was about 9:15 on a drizzly, grey, wet morning and I had just arrived at the elementary school, where, as an NP, I provide a weekly primary care clinic for the children who attend there, along with their families.

Two families were waiting in the hall for their appointments with me, and several more were hanging about hoping to see me that morning. The school secretary had a list of children who needed checking on for a variety of issues – from minor skin infections to sore throats, as well as a child who was vomiting and feverish. This was very typical. For so many families in this neighbourhood having access to health care at the school just made life simpler and less of a hassle.

I opened the door of my office, and began first by chatting to the "drop in families" to get a sense of urgency and then to start with my first scheduled family. The first hour raced by and I was about to call in the next family, when I noticed a petite, Spanish woman looking anxious in the hallway. She approached me shyly, looking uneasy, and asked to see me. I recognized her. I had met her very briefly twice before in my regular primary care clinic: once for a pregnancy test, and then again last week when she asked to make an appointment with me regarding her birth control concerns and her need for a regular health care provider for herself and her children. We had made an appointment for the following week for a full new patient visit. On both occasions our meetings had been brief, and I had found her very shy, polite and quite sad. At least that was my first impression.

It was quite chaotic there in the hallway. Children were running in and out, laughing and yelling, many young parents and toddlers hustling to attend a "mom and tot" program, and rambunctious noise was coming from the adjacent gymnasium. The hallway was certainly not a private place to ask what was wrong. I felt badly, as I told her I was full that morning, and I became more concerned when she became quite teary. Sensing her anxiety, I gave her the option of waiting for me or seeing one of my NP colleagues at another site. She made an attempt to wipe her tears, smiled weakly and sat down in the chair. I peeked out during the morning to see if she was still there. Each time she briefly glanced up and nodded at me. She waited almost two hours, sitting quietly, never moving from her place on the chair in the hallway.

When the clinic ended, I collected her and brought her into my school office and offered her tea, which she refused politely. Susanna was a petite, shy, Spanish woman, who was only in her twenties. She has three children, who were all pre-school age. I asked her how I could help her, which was my standard greeting. A tear trickled down her cheek and without looking up she told me that her support person had insisted that she come to my office—so she came. I placed my hand on her knee, and asked her once again what was wrong, and how could I help her.

She looked so sad and remained silent for several minutes. Finally, she looked at me and told me that she used to go to this school. Having allowed her to continue, she said that her husband had left her and had moved back to his homeland the previous week. “I don’t want to live anymore,” she said sadly.

The school bell rang, startling me, yet Susanna seemed to have not heard it. She didn’t move. I was conscious of the sounds of children running back into the school after the lunch break. The air was filled with their happy noise, yet inside the office, there was such sadness. Tears dripped down Susanna’s face. She began to talk again, telling me now that although he had gone, she sees him at night after the children have gone to bed. She said that she hears music in the house when there is no one home, and questioned whether she was losing her mind. She was desperate—and sad.

I was at a loss of what to say or do. I did not know Susanna well enough and had no knowledge of her medical history, and in a very non-clinical setting such as the school, I was scrambling as to how to proceed. She needed help—and urgently. The situation was complicated. She had three small children who were going to need picking up after their childcare programs ended that day. She seemed so alone.

I began asking about her children; they were eighteen months, three and four years old. I asked who would look after them if she could not, and I asked if she had a plan for harming herself. Susanna sat slumped in a chair, staring at her lap with her hair hiding much of her face, and throughout our conversation her voice was soft and monotone. Tears fell silently as she outlined her suicide plan and her belief that their father would have to come back to get them if she was dead. I performed a depression screen, which was strongly positive. I was not surprised, but I was querying an acute psychosis. I told her I needed to extract a promise from her that she would not harm herself, and her response was that she could not promise that, as she had nothing left.

She needed an urgent psychiatric referral so it appeared that I would have to call 911. I was concerned about the impact that this would have on Susanna, and also on the school staff and students of having an ambulance and police arrive at the school. I was worried about her young children and who could care for them. The situation was complex and very messy.

I made a call to the emergency department's psychiatric intake RN at our local hospital to assist with planning, as this was not a situation I had ever experienced previously. She made an urgent request to the psychiatrist on call who, after hearing my story, agreed with me that an urgent admission was needed and she would see Susanna as soon as she arrived at the emergency department. I could have hugged her! I wasn't alone! Then she explained that most likely Susanna would need a 4–6 week in-patient admission. *Good heavens,* I thought, *that's going to be a problem* – I did not want her to risk losing her children to the foster care system. I had learned from Susanna's counsellor that she was an excellent caring mother and she loved her children. Her family needed to remain intact somehow while she got well.

Susanna and I talked about the plan. I needed her to agree and to feel that someone cared, and that she would get help. I held her hand while we talked. She agreed to go to the hospital and, still holding her hand, I called 911 and gave the school address to the dispatcher. The next step was to find someone to help with the children, at least temporarily.

Susanna gave me permission to get in touch with her mother who lived in the neighbourhood, although she asked me not to tell her that she was going to see a psychiatrist as she was worried about being thought of as "crazy". As her mother did not speak much English, I needed some help with interpreting. The situation was becoming more complicated by the minute. Susanna called her mother, and she and a friend arrived at the school. The friend spoke English, so I told them that Susanna was ill and I was arranging for an ambulance to take her to the hospital, and that she might be there for a week or so. I hadn't spoken the full truth; however I had made a promise to Susanna, which ultimately was at this time, in the best interests for everyone. Her mother agreed to take the children, which would then give me time to sort out additional support for the grandmother and the children.

I could hear a disturbance outside the door of the office, and I was shocked when I opened the door to see the paramedics. They looked like police officers. Susanna was looking quite scared. After they completed their assessment and I was able to reassure her that she would be well cared for, I gave them an envelope with the documentation of my assessment for the psychiatrist. Once they had left I was totally shocked to acknowledge that the entire encounter had only taken ninety minutes – it felt like a lifetime!

I was amazed at the progress Susanna made toward recovery after that horrific encounter two years ago. Having been on antipsychotic medication she became more stable, however, still suffers occasionally from anxiety. She continues to see me on a monthly basis for active mental health monitoring, while moving closer to her extended family, and she has recently started a part-time job. Susanna has embraced the mental health counselling that I was able to arrange for her through a non-profit organization, and her children are healthy and beautiful.

Since that time, Susanna and her children are regular patients in my practice; it is so lovely to see the children grow, to watch her parenting style that is both strong and loving and to see her blossom. I asked her on one of her routine visits what prompted her to see me that day, and her response was that she had a good feeling . . . she knew that I would help her and the children. I have thought about her remark often and I think that it speaks volumes about the importance of the relationship that is established between the NP and the patient, without judgment or preconceived notions, and most of all with respect for the patient's life and beliefs.

For me, Susanna reminds me every time I see her of the resilience of our patients and their families, if we simply offer them a chance to succeed. I am always grateful over the course of my daily NP practice to be allowed into the lives of the families; it is this which gives me the greatest pleasure as an NP.

Maya's Moccasins

Anne Claire Desrosiers MN-NP (F)

Maya was not very loud or talkative. She sat in my office with her hands in her lap and looked down at the floor. She spoke softly and told me that she wanted to sew again. I did my best to find out why she had stopped sewing in the first place, and she told me that her hands hurt too much. Maya went on to tell me that not only did her hands hurt, but her feet hurt too. She was now finding it hard to walk, with pain in her feet and knees, and her lower back; however, on this particular day, it was the pain in her hands that had brought her to my office.

She went on to tell me that she needed to make moccasins. She was an Indigenous Elder in the community, and a member of the teaching staff in the town school. She was trying to maintain her sense of culture, and to continue teaching that culture to the children of her community and at the school. She needed to make moccasins.

I examined her hands and feet. She didn't have any palpable nodes, red, hot joints, loss of sensation or loss of range of motion. Maya said that her hands were at their worst in the morning, and when she tried to get out of bed she felt she couldn't even step on her feet, they were so painful. She explained how she would shuffle from her bedroom to the kitchen to make tea, and once she got going her feet would feel better. However, the pain would never completely go away. Her hands followed the same trajectory through the day. They would be stiff and sore in the morning but with some movement and with some use of them, the pain would abate a little as the day progressed. She continued to suffer through morning stiffness of her feet and hands, until one day she realized her baseline pain was so bad she couldn't pick up her leather awl to finish the moccasins she was working on. She needed to finish the moccasins; she needed to make more.

We agreed to do some screening blood work and that she could start taking pain medication regularly, and increase the dose if the pain was worsening. We agreed on a trial of pain medication until we could get the results of her blood work. I told her that the most likely diagnosis was inflammatory arthritis and explained the hallmark pathology of the disease. We talked about the relatives in her family that might have similar conditions or other inflammatory type diseases. Finally, I told her that this was a common ailment of the Indigenous population of the area; however, Maya informed me that this wasn't her country and that she was from the north. She went on to tell me that she had come from the Northwest Territories in her early twenties, and had been here for almost thirty years. I apologized for assuming that because she was First Nations she was local to the area. Maya thanked me for my time that day and left my office.

On the day I met Maya, I was working at a clinic I attended weekly. It was nearly a one-hour drive to the closest town in a very remote northern part of British Columbia. My colleague and I had been providing services there twice a week over the last four months. I was new to the profession. I had previously been working as a Registered Nurse for six years, with the bulk of my career in small community emergency departments here in Canada and in Australia. Although I was new to providing primary care, I was not unfamiliar with the challenges of rural and remote northern life.

Sure enough – as I had expected – Maya's blood work was positive for inflammatory markers. It was quite likely she had inflammatory arthritis. I contacted a rheumatologist who travelled throughout the province providing services in small towns where specialty medical services were not readily available. I was advised he would be able to see Maya during his next visit, which was almost eight weeks away. I asked if there was anything I could do for her in the meantime, if there was any further diagnostic testing to be done or medication she could try until he was able to see her himself. Dr. Stewart was more than pleased with my offer. He asked me to ensure she had an updated file, health history, medication list, and he asked me to order certain blood tests to have for him when he arrived. We discussed the trajectory of inflammatory arthritis care and potential issues that could arise when providing treatment. One of the best forms of treatment involved the use of immune suppressing drugs like methotrexate and biologic medications like adalimumab, both of which required some supervision. To minimize any potential side effects, we needed to ensure Maya was as healthy as possible before she could start either of those medications.

I asked Maya to return to the clinic a few weeks later. I informed her of the conversation that I'd had with Dr. Stewart and the trajectory of a disease like inflammatory arthritis. I explained the medications and asked if Maya could answer some questions about her health history to ensure we had all the information to make an informed choice.

Maya told me that she did not know her health history. She had no recollection of her mother or father and told me that she was taken to a residential school when she was five years old and stayed there until she was fifteen. She ran away and discovered the means to survive until she met the man she was going to marry, who brought her here when she was eighteen. Maya wouldn't discuss her time at residential school. She did, however, tell me that she had lost count of the times that she had been sick but was unaware of the reasons behind it. But her babies had been born well and were now healthy adults, which made her believe that any illness that she had had could not have been too bad. I asked Maya if I could contact the local health districts in the Northwest Territories to see if we could access her health files. She agreed.

For the remainder of her visit we reviewed the pain in her hands and feet. It seemed the over the counter medication, ibuprofen, was working for her. We agreed to continue the dose and added some strengthening exercises for her to do until she could see Dr. Stewart. Maya agreed to get the blood work done that he had requested, along with a chest x-ray. I called the public health unit in Yellowknife that day. After I explained what I was looking for, I was informed that any health files from the residential school might be at the new Indigenous Health Centre on the reserve on the other side of town. I was also advised the information I was looking for probably didn't exist, and if it did, it would not necessarily be easy to access. The federal government had already paid a visit to the health centre looking for files. The Indigenous Health Centre confirmed this; if Maya's information existed, there would be a legal battle for me to get it. Given the power of Maya's emotions around her life in the residential school, I did not push the issue with either health centre.

I called Dr. Stewart's office back. I asked what I should do about Maya's file, and about her immunization records. He referred me to the public health office and the centre for disease control for information. I formulated a plan with the information I gleaned from those offices and then I called Maya back to the office.

Maya told me that she was willing to do anything in order to make moccasins—whatever was needed. We agreed she would get further blood work done, to discover her immunity to several diseases she may have been exposed to. She agreed to have additional immunizations given based on that blood work.

We spent the next few weeks arranging and giving Maya her medications and immunizations. She finally got to see the rheumatologist, who promptly got her started on methotrexate, by weekly injection. Along with the nursing staff, Maya continued to see me regularly, and learned how to give herself the injections.

A few weeks later Maya told me that she was going to go on a trip to Arizona. She was taking some well-behaved children to the "healing lands". Maya wanted to know how she could take her injections on the plane with her for the two weeks she would be away. I called Dr. Stewart and we discussed the possibility of Maya switching to an oral version of methotrexate while she was away. We talked about the dosing and precautions and other medications. Dr. Stewart ordered a new oral medication and Maya went off to the desert. During her trip she did very well with her oral medication, and remained so during the summer.

Maya started to sew again and had completed a pair of moccasins. She thanked me and I responded by telling her that it had been my pleasure to help her.

Maya still comes to see me; we have worked through a number of health issues that she and her family have faced. Co-ordinating Maya's care and medical interventions with a specialist may have been par for the course in the career of an NP, yet, having the ability to help her was an extraordinary human experience I will never forget.

Mental Health Blending into Physical Symptoms

Elizabeth Sofia Berlin
(Family Nurse Practitioner)

One of the first patients I saw at our newly established hospital-based NP clinic in our rural northern town was Steve. Steve was a twenty-five-year old married logger with a life-long history of anxiety. This guy could have written the book on anxiety; in fact, his therapist Stacie had tapped into his knowledge by having him help her teach a life-skills program on coping with anxiety. He was a very intelligent man, and very self-aware. The issue that drove him to my clinic was a five-month bout of nausea that resulted in a twenty-pound weight loss. At his heaviest, Steve had only ever been 135 pounds, so this amount was very concerning to him.

Over the previous six months, he had been to our local community medical clinic a number of times, and had seen several different physicians. He felt that the physicians were extremely dismissive of his health concerns, chalking them all up to anxiety. This kind of treatment angered him, and he felt discriminated against because of his mental health issues, so much so that in the beginning, he would start each appointment with me discussing his experience and that he would never be going "up there" again. Steve had researched his symptoms online thoroughly, and had arrived with a number of possible diagnoses – lymphoma, a thyroid issue, and Crohn's disease, to name a few. He also had a pretty good idea which tests he felt should be ordered to determine if one of these might be the culprit.

Our first appointment lasted forty minutes, during which time Steve mostly shared his story. However, my NP brain broke it down into his chief complaint, history of present illness, past medical history, social history, and family medical history. I provided him with a lab requisition for blood tests, and asked him to come back the following week to review his test results and for a full physical examination. He also signed a consent form to have his complete medical records transferred to my clinic, and I accepted his request to become his Primary Health Care Provider.

Steve returned the following week as I'd suggested. The lab results helped us determine that his thyroid function was normal, but there were some strange things going on with his blood counts. His physical examination revealed some mild tenderness over his stomach, and the weight loss had us both very concerned. Most alarming to me was that his symptoms had been left unchecked for so long.

In our tiny community, my NP students are always blown away by the lack of primary health care – people often have to wait two or three weeks to see their family doctor. As NPs, we are also very busy, though it is rare to wait more than a week to see us. All of the physicians rotate in and out of the town – usually on a two weeks in, two weeks out arrangement; none of them reside here full time. You can imagine the breakdown of care this creates. My colleague and I generally see several new patients a day who start their appointment with, "I'm here today because Dr. X is unavailable for the next three weeks and this just can't wait." However, access to a specialty consultation is quite easy once the practitioner is aware of all of the resources available. One of these is the "RACE" line – a phone line with access to various on-call medical specialists, including a cardiologist, rheumatologist, oncologist, and gastroenterologist, among others. We also have several visiting specialists to our community and also have specialists available at some of the larger surrounding centres to which we can refer our patients.

One week after our initial appointment, and two appointments later, I had read through Steve's medical record, perused his blood work, and completed a full physical exam. My biggest fear was that this young man was wasting away from cancer, and his blood work suggested as much. I called the RACE line and was connected with an oncologist at the cancer centre for the north within minutes. Fortunately, his expertise allowed him to reassure me that the picture was not as bleak as it seemed to me. He offered to remain involved in his case, and suggested I order a CT scan of Steve's abdomen and chest to fully rule out a cancerous mass, and to do a test for tuberculosis.

My next plan was to refer Steve on an urgent basis to a gastroenterologist to help sort out his symptoms of nausea and lack of appetite. The oncologist I had spoken with on the RACE line had offered to consult with the gastroenterologist after she had seen Steve, so that they could work together on the case. Things progressed fairly quickly from there and Steve – despite his ongoing weight loss – was thrilled with the care he was receiving. He came in almost weekly, as his anxiety was high. Most of my care at that stage was reassurance, explaining the processes involved in having the various tests done that I had ordered for him, and reviewing possible diagnoses with him that he had printed off various internet websites. He continued to see his mental health therapist and psychiatrist regularly regarding the anxiety as well.

The CT scans and tuberculosis test were reassuring, showing only mild inflammation in his colon. While waiting to see the gastroenterologist – a wait of six weeks – he dipped to a low of 97 pounds. Also during that time, he developed a boil over his tailbone, which was really distressing to him. The gastroenterologist I had referred Steve to was a woman I had met at a presentation on celiac disease, which she had given recently. She was incredibly well spoken, intelligent, and personable. Steve and his wife had to drive several hours in order to see her. She personally performed a colonoscopy and endoscopy that day in her office – that is, used a tube with a small camera to thoroughly explore his bowels from top to bottom. She also took biopsies (samples of tissue) to make sure the mucous linings were healthy. She started him on a medication based on the results of the CT that we had had done, and sent me a full report of her findings while we awaited the biopsy results.

Steve came in that following week to debrief about that consultation. While his wife was equally impressed with this specialist, Steve felt that again his symptoms were being "swept under the rug" of his anxiety. He had brought detailed notes listing all of his symptoms to his appointment with the gastroenterologist, and she was not interested in reading these. I reassured him that she was not being dismissive in this case, that she had thoroughly investigated his symptoms. Indeed, he had gained several pounds on the medication she had prescribed, and the boil on his tailbone had healed. Physically, things were finally on the upswing. Once the biopsy results were back, Steve went to discuss the results with the gastroenterologist. Surprisingly to all of us, his gastrointestinal tract was completely healthy. The inflammation noted on the CT was not seen on the tests which had been performed.

During the second visit to the gastroenterologist, she reassured Steve there was absolutely no physical reason for his symptoms of nausea and weight loss. The changes on blood work that I had noted initially had normalized, and were likely due to a viral illness that had now resolved. Thus, the explanation for all of these issues could be traced back to the anxiety. Of course, her consultations were sent back to me as Steve's primary health care provider, as well as to his therapist and psychiatrist.

With renewed emphasis on appropriate management of his anxiety through medication and mental health therapy, Steve's weight slowly climbed back up to 115 pounds. He continued to come in regularly to discuss his plans to return to work, to attempt to reintroduce a variety of foods, and the progress with his anxiety management. Three months after our initial visit, Steve's weight was back to baseline, we had fully ruled out all physical causes of his symptoms, and he was on a gradual return to work plan.

Discrimination in health care is a very real issue. In our northern British Columbia community, we regularly hear our patients' concerns that they have experienced racism and discrimination based on their weight, poverty, or mental health concerns within the health care system. The psychiatrist visits our community monthly to help co-manage patients with mental health issues. These patients generally are linked with one of our two Mental Health Therapists. The patients also have a Primary Health Care Provider – either an NP or a family physician. The collaboration among members of this team is essential to providing high quality health care for this often vulnerable and marginalized group. While in the process of sorting out physical symptoms for a young schizophrenic patient that I co-manage with the psychiatrist, I phoned the psychiatrist to discuss whether the issue was physical, mental or both. The psychiatrist told me that earlier that week one of his patients had died of a "schizophrenic bowel cancer", meaning he had died of the cancer, but it had not been properly investigated because of discrimination around his mental health issue.

As NPs, we are grounded in the profession of nursing. Nurses advocate for their patients in all manner of settings, including hospital and home and community care. We are experts at navigating the health care system in order to help our patients understand the confusing journey through diagnostic testing and results. We are embedded in the communities we serve and soundly networked with the resources available to our patients. We assist our patients to construct the appropriate team of professionals, volunteers, and community agencies and resources to help meet their individual needs and build on the capacities they have. These are just a few of the components of added value that nurses bring to the role of primary health care provider.

No One Left Behind

Final thoughts from the Author

This book was written to answer the question: "What do nurse practitioners do?" It is my hope this collection of true stories from NPs across Canada has provided some powerful insight into that question. As the most studied group of health professionals in history, we have a vast amount of data describing the value which NPs bring to the health care system. Research alone, however, cannot capture the true depths of the work we do and the impact we have on patients. Only by sharing our stories can we hope to fully articulate our role.

Perhaps because of our history and the evolution of the NP role in Canada, NPs have learned to stick together, to support each other, to celebrate our victories and weep together at our losses. We prop each other up when it is most needed, in a manner I believe is unique among other professions. We leave none of our colleagues behind.

The NP role evolved from the need to provide health care to those who need it most, those who are most isolated, both geographically and socially. In our efforts to ensure all Canadians receive the necessary health care,

NPs have gone where few others have gone before. And we will continue to do so, pushing the boundaries of health policy and challenging the status quo, until all Canadians can access the health care they need, no matter where they live.

We will leave no one behind.

Claudia Mariano

About the Contributors

Michelle Acorn DNP, NP PHC/Adult, ENC(C), GNC(C), holds dual Nurse Practitioner specialty certifications in Primary Health Care and Adult. She is a Past President of the Nurse Practitioner Association of Ontario. Michelle is the Lead NP at the NP-led model of care at Lakeridge Health Hospital in Whitby, Ontario. She is also the Primary Health Care-Global Health Coordinator and lecturer at the University of Toronto. Michelle Co-chairs the Central East Local Health Integration Network Health Professions Advisory Council & the RNAO/NPAO Hospital Toolkit Expert Advisory Group. Michelle successfully innovated multiple NP Models of care to date. Michelle has been awarded the Jerry Gerow NP Leadership Award, Lakeridge Awards of Excellence, Fleming Alumni of Distinction & Preceptor of the Year Award. She is also a Queen's Silver Jubilee and Premier's Award Nominee. Michelle is a principal and site investigator/researcher for NP scholarship, with a special interest in Most Responsible Provider (MRP).

Elizabeth Berlin Family Nurse Practitioner, lives in British Columbia on the shores of Burns Lake with her husband, and two sons, aged seven and four. She worked as a Community Health Nurse in First Nations communities for eight years prior to completing her Masters as Family Nurse Practitioner with the University of Northern British

Columbia in 2010. She and her colleague, Anne Desrosiers, also featured in this book, share a busy family practice in the Lakes District of Northern BC. They provide NP clinics at the local hospital, as well as five outreach clinics that include several First Nations communities. Presently, she is also serving a two year term as the Northern Health Authority representative for the British Columbia Nurse Practitioners' Association. She enjoys gardening, organic cooking, sewing, and exploring the great outdoors through running, hiking, cycling, and cross country skiing.

Kate Burkholder MN, NP, is a nurse practitioner who works in the small rural fishing community of Black's Harbour New Brunswick. She was one of the first Nurse Practitioners to practice in New Brunswick in this new role for nurses in 2003. She lives in St Stephen, New Brunswick with her husband, with her two daughters and their families and two grandchildren, and mother nearby. It is a close knit family. She has chaired and been a member of various provincial and national committees related to the many aspects of Nurse Practitioner practice. After 38 years in nursing and 12 as a Nurse Practitioner, Kate describes the nurse practitioner role as one of the most rewarding roles for nurses as "we weave through people's lives; integrating our clinical skills, knowledge of research, and evidence based practice with the love for our community and the strength of the supports within them. What better a role can a nurse fulfill? I always said nursing was about caring, competence and compassion and I feel as an NP I do this every day; it is a win-win."

Marilyn Butcher NP-PHC, co-authored the proposal for the first NP led clinic in Canada and retired from her position as inaugural Clinic Director in 2010. She remains on the Board of Directors of the Sudbury District NP Clinic.

Marilyn has launched her own consulting firm to work with health care organizations, including NP – Led clinics. She has co- authored several articles regarding primary health care reform in Canada. Marilyn has been an active member of the Registered Nurses' Association of Ontario and the Nurse Practitioners' Association of Ontario, and was given an Honourary Lifetime Award from NPAO and a Lawrence S. Bloomberg Faculty of Nursing Award of Distinction from the University of Toronto.

Anne Desrosiers MN-NP(F), graduated from the University of British Columbia Master's Nursing-Nurse Practitioner program in 2013 after a four year career in nursing and a three year career in teaching. She holds a Bachelor of Health Sciences from the University of Western Ontario which she applied in her teaching career in rural Georgia, US. She came to nursing with the pride and immense support of her family, as she is the fourth generation trained as a nurse and third generation practicing nurse. Her nursing career brought her to many different communities throughout Canada and Australia and she is currently practicing primary health care as a Nurse Practitioner in rural northern British Columbia. Her next move is to Scotland to be with her partner and explore even more nursing opportunities.

Kathryn Flanigan MN, NP-PHC, graduated from the University of Toronto in 1986 with her Bachelor of Science in Nursing. She completed her PHC-NP certificate in 1999 from Western University then returned to complete her Master of Nursing degree in 2013. Kathryn was the recipient of the 2013-2014 Elizabeth Wooster Gold Medal Award for highest academic standing in the MScN/MN program at Western. She has worked for nine years at a Community

Health Centre in Kitchener, Ontario. She is currently working as a nurse practitioner in primary health care at an academic Family Health Team, where she also participates in research and presents on practice issues to support clinical practice. Kathryn has received Level 1 certification in Pelvic Health Rehabilitation.

Donna Kearney MHS, NP-PHC, grew up in rural Ontario and developed a passion for delivering healthcare to rural communities. She became a RN in 1988 after completing the diploma program at the British Columbia Institute of Technology, and went on to pursue a Bachelor of Science in Nursing degree, a Bachelor of Arts in Gerontology, and the Nurse Practitioner Certificate at Laurentian University, completed in 2003. She was extremely fortunate to be offered the position of starting a nursing station in Rosseau, Ontario; a job she often refers to as the best NP job in all of Ontario! In 2008, she completed an online Master's in Health Studies - Leadership Stream from Athabasca University. Currently, she works as a consultant at the company she founded, Rural Health Solutions, to develop rural health delivery strategies. It is also her great privilege to teach in the NP Program through Queen's University in Ontario.

Charlotte McCallum MN, NP-Adult, GDipNPAC is a nurse practitioner in the department of Anesthesia and Perioperative Medicine, and an Adjunct Assistant Professor at the Arthur Labatt Family School of Nursing at Western University in London, Ontario. Charlotte's professional work and prior national specialty certifications include critical care, neurosciences, and nephrology nursing. Additional professional activities include national nursing specialty exam development, guest lecturing, project consultation, and health advocacy. As a Nurse Practitioner, Charlotte has clinical experience in intensive care, hemodialysis and complex pain. Charlotte is passionate about nursing professional activities, and innovative health care system changes to optimize the health of Ontarians and Canadians.

Calvin Pelletier NP-PHC, CHPCN(C) is a lifelong resident of Thunder Bay, Ontario, where he lives with his beautiful wife and energetic seven year old daughter. After completing degrees in biochemistry and nursing at Lakehead University, he attended the University of Manitoba for the Intensive Care Nursing Program. After completing his program he travelled to Canada's north, where he worked for eight years, during which time he completed a Management Program through McMaster University. After the birth of their daughter the Pelletier Family returned to Thunder Bay where he returned to Lakehead University and completed the Nurse Practitioner Program. Calvin currently works at the local Community Care Access Centre as a Primary Health Care Nurse Practitioner in Palliative Care, where he is involved in several chronic disease and pain management programs. Calvin has continued on with palliative care education, completing a De Sousa course in Palliative Care as well as a Canadian Nurses' Association certification in palliative care. Calvin is an active board member on many professional advisory committees.

Natasha Prodan-Bhalla MN/NP (A), DNP(c) is an Adult Nurse Practitioner in Vancouver, British Columbia. She graduated with a Bachelor of Science in Nursing degree from the University of Western Ontario and an MN/NP degree from the University of Toronto. Natasha worked for many years on a post-operative cardiac surgery unit and is currently working on her Doctor of Nursing Practice (DNP) at University of Colorado. She is an adjunct professor at the University of

British Columbia and the University of Victoria. Her current practice focus is women's health that includes leading a primary prevention heart program for women and working in a primary health clinic for marginalized women. Her story reflects the passion she feels about being a Nurse Practitioner and how honored she is to have the opportunity to develop such strong and significant relationships with her patients.

Kathryn Roka NP-PHC was a law clerk at Toronto-based law firms Osler Hoskin & Harcourt and McMillan Binch for 12 years specializing in bankruptcy and insolvency law. Making a career change from law to nursing in 2003, Kathryn graduated from York University (BScN) and worked for Peterborough Health Department - High Risk Pediatric Health for five years. In 2008, Kathryn graduated from Queen's University as a Primary Health Care Nurse Practitioner. She has worked in a variety of PHC settings and maintains NP registration in Ontario and Prince Edward Island. Kathryn is the NPAO Director of Education since 2012 and founder and past chair of the Durham Region NP Group. She is currently pursuing graduate studies at Queen's University with hopes to move into PhD stream in 2016.

Lorine Scott MN, NP (F) completed her MN NP (F) program at the University of Victoria in 2005 after a career in nursing spanning over 30 years. She is currently a Family Nurse Practitioner at the BC Children's Hospital in the capacity of Primary Care Lead with the RICHER Initiative, an innovative inner city health care outreach program. As co-lead she was responsible for the development and implementation of the Responsive Intersectoral/Interdisciplinary Child/Community Health Education & Research Initiative (RICHER), a program that "takes health care to hard to reach families in the inner city". This practice and research initiative, the first of its kind in BC was awarded a Health Canada Innovations Award in 2012. As co-investigator, Lorine has co-authored 4 peer reviewed articles related to this model of health care delivery and provided numerous lectures related to serving marginalized/vulnerable children and families. Championing the NP role she continues to provide professional leadership as adjunct faculty at the University of British Columbia School of Nursing, Chair of the College of Registered Nurses of British Columbia Nurse Practitioner Exam Committee, and has served two previous terms as President of the British Columbia Nurse Practitioner Association. She has two children and three grandchildren and a supportive partner who shares in her achievements.

Marnee Wilson MSc, NP-Adult, CDE has provided care to patients with cardiovascular disease throughout her nursing career. She has been a Nurse Practitioner since 2000 and obtained specialty certification in the Adult Class when the first exam was available in Ontario after the title protection legislation was passed in 2007. She is the Professional Practice Leader for Nurse Practitioners at St. Michael's Hospital in Toronto and works clinically with cardiac surgical patients at St. Michael's Hospital. She is an Adjunct Lecturer and Course Instructor at the University of Toronto, the Director of Professional Practice at the Nurse Practitioners' Association of Ontario, and leads a Community of Practice for hospital-based NPs. Marnee has worked with numerous hospitals in Ontario to facilitate full implementation of the NP role. She has received numerous awards and recognitions, including the Jerry Gerow Award from the Nurse Practitioners' Association of Ontario, for outstanding contribution to the association and development of the NP role.

About the Author

Claudia Mariano is a Primary Health Care Nurse Practitioner from Ontario, Canada, with twenty-nine years of experience as a registered nurse and nurse practitioner, working with some of the most vulnerable patients. Former president of the Nurse Practitioners' Association of Ontario, she has presented at numerous professional conferences on a variety of health care topics.

After obtaining her undergraduate degree in Nursing from the University of Toronto 1986, Claudia returned to the University of Toronto and obtained her Master of Science degree in 1992. In 1999 she obtained her Primary Health Care Nurse Practitioner designation, also through the University of Toronto. Claudia is also a Certified Diabetes Educator. For the past seven years she has worked at a Family Health Team in Pickering and prior to that she worked at a Community Health Centre in Toronto for ten years, working with marginalized populations.

Claudia resides with her husband and three sons in Pickering, Ontario, close to the shores of Lake Ontario.

www.ingramcontent.com/pod-product-compliance
Lightning Source LLC
Chambersburg PA
CBHW021954170526
45157CB00003B/990